Protect Yourself from Violence

Tactics, Tools and Preparations

George A. DeFillipo

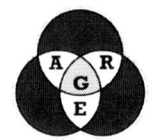

Arge Publishing
P.O. Box 492863
Redding, Ca 96049
protectyourselffromviolence.com

Copyright © 2013 Arge Publishing – George A. DeFillipo
All rights reserved.

Except for brief excerpts in a review, no part of this book shall be reproduced, stored in any retrieval system, or transmitted by electronic, mechanical, photocopying, or any other means, including posting on the internet and other forms of distribution, without written permission from the publisher. Violations are illegal and punishable by law.

ISBN 978-0-9910128-0-0
Library of Congress Catalog Number 2013956356

Agent/Project Manager: Penny Callmeyer,
Tiger Lilly Enterprises

Cover and Text Design/Layout: Jason O. Crye

Attention:
Contact the publisher for information on quantity discounts.

Printed and bound in the United States of America
at Color House Graphics, Grand Rapids, Michigan

First Edition December 2013

Author and Publisher Disclaimer

Although every precaution has been taken to insure the accuracy of the information in this book, the author assumes no responsibility for errors or omissions.

The information provided in this book is about personal protection. Defense against violent attack is by its nature inherently risky. Neither the author nor publisher can be held responsible for any injury, loss, damage or legal expenses allegedly relating to the use or misuse of the information provided.

It is impossible for a book to list all possible self-defense scenarios that can arise; therefore the reader is responsible for making his or her own sound judgments and good decisions.

The reader is responsible for being aware of and obeying all local, state and federal laws relating to self-defense, reasonable force and the use of weapons. We do not condone illegal activities of any kind. Nothing in this book should be construed as legal advice.

The mentioning of specific products by name are not necessarily recommendations for the purchase of these products to the exclusion of alternatives available. They are mentioned to provide the reader with concrete examples that can be viable choices. There are many products not mentioned in this book that would also make perfectly good alternatives to those provided and their exclusion does not in any manner lessen their viability. It is the responsibility of the reader to research which products available would best meet his or her needs. The author takes no responsibility for the performance of any product or service mentioned in this book.

The material is provided for academic study only.

Acknowledgements

First and foremost I would like to thank Professor Jane Carr, 9th Degree Black Belt, American Judo and Jujitsu Federation, for teaching me Modern Arnis. I am deeply indebted to her for teaching me this wonderful Filipino martial art where I have learned so much about the use of sticks and knives in self-defense. Professor Carr is co-author of the book, *Anatomy For Martial Artists*.

I would like to thank Scott Redden, 5th Degree Black belt, America Judo and Jujitsu Federation, 6th Degree Black Belt, American Practical Arnis, and author of the book, *Opening Your Mind With Martial Arts*, for his feedback, especially with subject content and sequence. I would also like to thank Stan Lundahl, 3rd Degree Black Belt, American Practical Arnis, for his many helpful suggestions, especially with content flow. Special thanks to Marilyn Traugott, 3rd Degree Black Belt, American Practical Arnis, for her astute editing suggestions.

I am most appreciative of Jered Hallstrom, Brown Belt, American Practical Arnis and former firearms professional, for his valuable input on guns and assistance with firearm photographs. Also, special thanks to Ron Kibler for his excellent firearms photographs.

I am very appreciative of Kung Fu Expert and friend, John L. Price, author of the book, *Masters Manual of Hsing-I Kung Fu*, for his helpful, candid input and suggestions.

I am grateful for the helpful suggestions that my friend Ray Mills has provided. His extensive military experience has made him more acutely aware of situational dangers of any person that I know.

I would like to express my gratitude to Dana Leigh Shafman, of Shieldher Inc., for teaching me about Tasers® and stun guns. Her expertise greatly enriched the information on this subject.

I would like to give thanks to my wife, Arlene, long-time Hsing-I Kung Fu practitioner, for her numerous suggestions and for patiently editing the manuscript of this book.

I would like to give special thanks to Robert W. Young, Executive Editor, *Black Belt* magazine, for granting me permission to reprint his outstanding editorial, "WHY SO MANY MARTIAL ARTISTS OPPOSE MORE GUN CONTROL" (see appendix A).

And my most sincere appreciation goes to Jason Crye for the creation of this book's outstanding cover and layout and publishing company logo.

Lastly, I would like to thank my Project Manager, Penny Callmeyer, with Tiger Lilly Enterprises, for her indispensible expertise and guidance. Her suggestions have significantly helped me to prepare this book for publication.

"Let us speak courteously, deal fairly, and keep ourselves armed and ready."

President Theodore Roosevelt
San Francisco, California
May 13, 1903

Table of Contents

Preface i
Introduction iii
Your Right To Self-Defense v

PART I: TACTICS

Violence – Just How Bad Is It Out There? 3
Criminals and You 7
The "AAA" Survival Concept 9
The Importance of Situational Awareness 11
Avoiding Trouble 15
Preparing for Trouble 17
Your Survival Mentality 19
Self-Defense Decisions 21

PART II: TOOLS

Self-Defense Options 25
Why You Should Carry a Weapon 27
Guns – The Great Equalizer 29
Knives – When You Don't Have a Gun 41

The Power of Impact Weapons 65
Other Tools for Self-Defense. 67
Martial Arts, Boxing, Wrestling And Other
Self-Defense Hand-To-Hand Fighting Systems 73

PART III: PREPARATIONS

The Value of Training 79
Self-Defense Seminars for Women. 83
Security in Your Home, Workplace & Vehicle 85
Especially Dangerous Places and Situations. 97
Legal Considerations. 103
How Do You Rate Being Safe?. 107
Conclusion 113

*Appendix A: "WHY SO MANY MARTIAL
ARTISTS OPPOSE GUN CONTROL"* 115
Appendix B: Where to Find Quality Training 121
Glossary 125
Recommended Reading 127
About the Author 133

Preface

I have written this book because I see an increasing need in our society for realistic self-defense. Crime is increasing in frequency, as is the severity of violence. As I write this book there have been two separate incidents during one week where local police officers have been brutally attacked during routine activities. In October of 2011, the murder of a family friend and seven others at his place of work in Seal Beach, California made national news. Crime is getting closer to home.

In addition, current tight budgets have resulted in reduced police services and more criminals being let out on the street. Unfortunately many people seem to be oblivious as to what is going on around them. I would like to see that change. I would like to see more people being aware of potential dangers in their lives and learn how they can realistically protect themselves if the need were to arise.

This book has been written to provide useful information on the topic of how to be safe from criminal violence. The information presented will provide the reader with a knowledge framework and practical advice. It has been written concise so that the fundamentals involved in being safe will not be lost in endless technical information. *Protect Yourself From Violence: Tactics, Tools And Preparations* is a helpful guide for those wanting to better protect themselves.

Everyone has a right and obligation to protect themselves and their families. It is an individual's natural right. The police cannot be everywhere; therefore your need for personal safety ultimately lies in your own hands. This book will discuss the various options available, including weapons and other tools that will assist you in keeping safe.

Introduction

No single way of protecting yourself is foolproof. What this book offers is the knowledge that a person needs to minimize the risk of being a victim of criminal attack. It also offers insight into the various tools available for self-defense and why I strongly recommend that you always have at least one with you.

Not being a victim begins with awareness. Awareness of the criminal mindset, awareness of situational dangers and awareness of what you are willing to do to defend yourself if attacked.

Fully protecting yourself includes being secure in your home, car, and workplace, as well as when traveling. Preparations you can take in each of these areas will be addressed in this book. I will provide reasons why specialized self-defense seminars are a very good idea for women, regardless of age. Lastly, I will address how you can minimize risk to yourself and your loved ones when in dangerous situations and places.

Your Right To Self-Defense

The following quotes are provided to show that you have a right to be able to defend yourself. Throughout the history of mankind, this right has been successfully defended many times. When taken away, it has resulted in needless suffering and death for millions of people.

"I refer to the law which lays it down that, if our lives are endangered by plots or violence or armed robbers or enemies, any and every method of protecting ourselves is morally right."

Cicero
Selected Political Speeches

"(Such a prince, he explained, would found his state upon) good laws and good arms. And as there cannot be good laws where there are not good arms, and where there are good arms there must be good laws, I will not now discuss the laws, but will speak of the arms."

Machiavelli
The Prince

"For those that possess and can wield arms are in a position to decide whether the constitution is to continue or not."

Aristotle
Politics

"Who does not see that self-defense is a duty superior to every precept (of personal freedom)."

Montesquieu
The Spirit of Laws

"A Covenant not to defend myself from force, by force, is always void. For…no man can transfer or lay down his Right to save himself from Death."

Thomas Hobbes
Leviathan

"Let your gun therefore be the constant companion of your walks."
"No Free man shall ever be debarred the use of arms."

President Thomas Jefferson
Papers of Thomas Jefferson

"Arms in the hands of citizens (may) be used at individual discretion…in private self-defense."

President John Adams
A Defense of the Constitutions of Government of the United States of America

"…arms…discourage and keep the invader and plunderer in awe, and preserve order in the world as well as property… Horrid mischief would ensue were (the law-abiding) deprived the use of them… The weak will become prey to the strong."

Thomas Paine
Writings of Thomas Paine

"The most foolish mistake we could possibly make would be to allow the subjected people to carry arms; history shows that all conquerors who have allowed their subjected people to carry arms have prepared their own fall."

Adolph Hitler
Edict of March 18, 1938

"Among the many misdeeds of the British rule in India, history will look upon the Act depriving a whole nation of arms as the blackest."

Mahatma Gandhi
*An Autobiography of the Story of
My Experiments with the Truth*

PROTECT YOURSELF FROM VIOLENCE

Part I
Tactics

Violence — Just How Bad Is It Out There?

It seems like everyday we get bombarded with news stories of incredible violence occurring; murderers torturing and decapitating their victims, random knife attacks on innocent people and violent rapes to name but a few. Is violent crime as bad as it appears in the news media or is it being sensationalized to get our attention and sell the news?

To get a better idea of what the reality is regarding violence, let's look at some statistics. In 2010, the U.S. Census Bureau reported that there were 308,745,538 people living in the United States. During that same year the Federal Bureau of Investigation reported in their Uniform Crime Report (the UCR) that there were 1,246,248 reported and verified violent crimes. These crimes break down into the following categories: 14,748 murders, 84,767 forcible rapes, 367,832 robberies and 778,901 aggravated assaults.

To make matters worse, it is estimated that only 40% of all violent crime is reported[1]. Often the victims are embarrassed, fearful or just don't believe it to be worthwhile reporting the crime to the police. So the real numbers are estimated to be more than 3 million violent crimes in 2010!

---

1 http://www.sociologyindex.com/measure_of_crime.htm

If other types of crimes (also reported by the FBI in their UCR report) such as property crimes, vehicle theft, burglary and larceny are included, you can add another 18 million plus crimes in 2010. This amounts to almost 20 million *reported* crimes for a population of approximately 300 million people. As the various law enforcement agencies use different terminologies for a crime, they can get categorized differently with some crime rates actually being reported artificially low.

The UCR measure of crime shows that over the 50-year period from 1960 to 2010 the number of violent crimes has increased approximately 430% while the population has increased approximately 72% (the 1960 United States population was 179,323,175 and violent crime was 288,460). In 1960 the violent crime rate was 160.9 per 100,000 people. In 2010 it was 403.6 per 100,000 people. In 2010 you were 2.5 times more likely to be a victim of violent crime than in 1960! Lastly, imprisonment rates have increased 200% over the last twenty years.[2]

I have pointed out the statistics of violent crime during one year, 2010. Multiply these numbers over a period of say 20 years and you will have a better appreciation of the likelihood that you or a family member may become a victim in the future. Obviously the numbers shoot way up and many people can expect to have a family member be the victim of a violent assault or experience an attempted assault.

There have been a number of studies and crime statistics that show a relationship between crime and drug use, poverty, and a lack of educational or employment opportunities. These studies show that crime goes up when there is poverty

---

2   Ibid.

and when the opportunities to find work are diminished. Since the economic crisis of late 2007-2008, many people have lost their jobs and homes and it is prudent for people to be prepared for continued increases in crime. It is not far-fetched to see crime sky rocket if economic conditions in the United States do not improve.

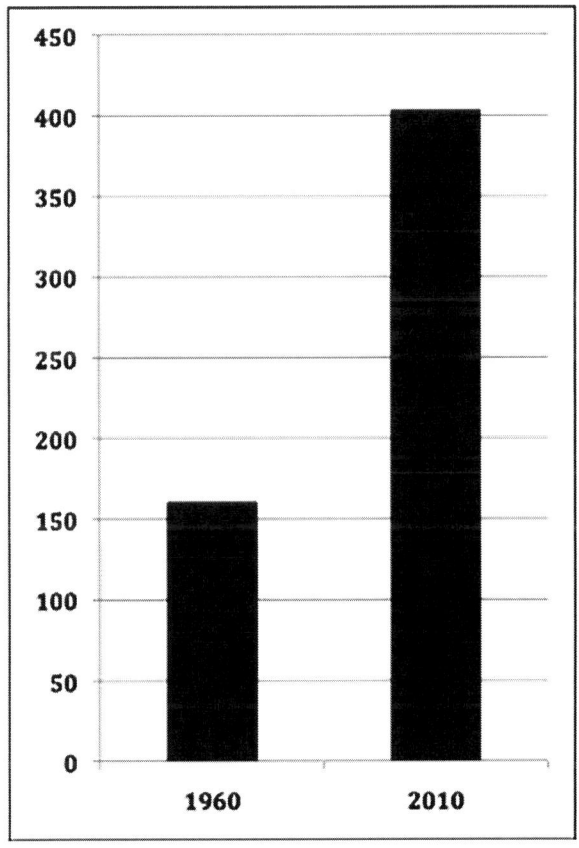

Chart shows rate increase of violent crime per 100,000 people in the United States.

PROTECT YOURSELF FROM VIOLENCE

Criminals and You

To a criminal you are not a human being with qualities to be valued. They don't care about your feelings or about your loved ones. Simply stated, they don't care about you. You are an object that they can murder, rob, assault or rape as the situation allows. The use of force to get their way is a given.

If criminals cared about others they wouldn't be criminals. Many criminals enjoy hurting others. They do so because they are emotionally damaged as human beings. Don't expect sympathy from them.

If a criminal plans to commit a crime, that criminal has already desensitized himself or herself to caring about you. You are just a means to getting what he or she wants. It is not uncommon for criminals to use degrading words and terms to describe their potential victims such as bitch, rich bastard or some racial degrading insult. This mentally helps them to justify their criminal behavior. Don't think that you can get them to be reasonable and leave you alone. You are most probably wasting your breath. What you can expect from a criminal is that they will not treat you fairly.

Their means of attack can include surprising or ambushing you, using multiple attackers, the use of weapons, etc. Occasionally, they will stand out in appearance, but many times they will look just like everyone else.

What most criminals like to do is look for easy victims. If you appear unaware of what's going on around you, weak, unable to defend yourself, and have something that they want, then consider yourself fair game.

To survive you must be willing to do what it takes to not be a victim. You must learn to not be vulnerable. And you must have a strong will to win if you are attacked.

The first thing that you need to do is not stand out. That means not standing out in any way. You want to blend in with everyone else. How you dress and what car you drive can make you look like a potential victim to a criminal. Let's stop for a moment and try to think like a criminal. If you were a criminal wouldn't you like to find someone who looks vulnerable. Someone who looks soft from the street point of view and probably can be "set-up" in some way. Someone who is oblivious as to what is around them. And wouldn't you as a criminal like to find prey that has nice things such as clothing, jewelry or an expensive car? In other words, someone a criminal deems worth robbing, raping or assaulting.

The point that I am making is the less that you look like prey, the less likely that you will be preyed upon. Don't stand out as a victim.

The other part of the prey equation is to not look like an easy victim. You want to look like you can take care of yourself; that you are not to be messed with.

The "AAA" Survival Concept

I would like to introduce you to the "AAA" Survival Concept. These are the big three components involved in not being a victim. Each of these three components begins with the letter A, and together make up the "AAA" survival concept. They are **Awareness**, **Avoidance** and **Armed**. These are the key components of coming home intact. Getting good at them will significantly improve your chances of not being a victim.

Each of these key components will be discussed and explained in future chapters of this book.

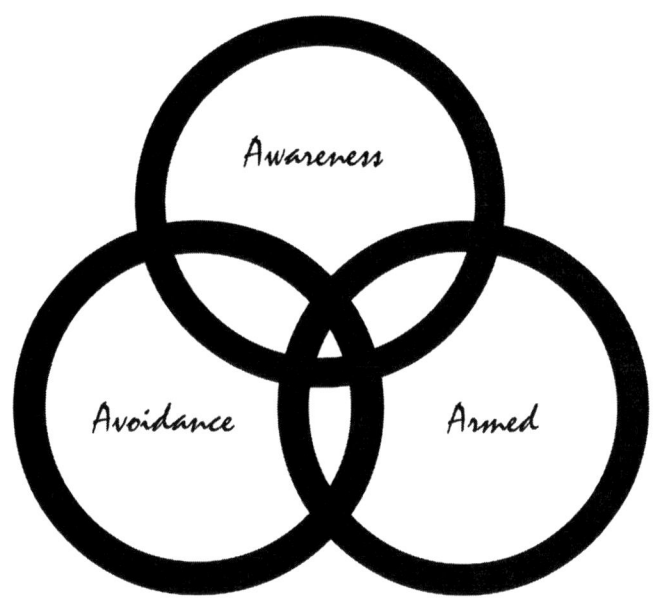

"AAA" SURVIVAL CONCEPT

The Importance of Situational Awareness

The human body is wired for fight or flight when confronted by dangerous situations. Being aware of your immediate environment or the environment that you are possibly going into can save you from having to deal with a dangerous situation. It can also give you the time to better deal with a dangerous situation that you may not have time to avoid altogether.

You need to get into the habit of being aware of what is going on around you at all times. Don't worry about what other people might think of you. Your safety is more important. It is perfectly all right to be scanning ahead and to your sides as you proceed forward, making sure that there is no potential danger that could come near you. It is also wise to occasionally glance over your shoulder to make sure that no one is back there that shouldn't be. You are not being paranoid. You are being smart.

I like to use a version of the four-level color code system to measure different levels of awareness and danger. The first level is called condition **CODE WHITE**. When a person is in condition code white they are not aware of their surroundings at all. They are totally engulfed in some activity such as being in deep thought, talking, playing or reading. People in condition code white are oblivious of any potential dangers.

They are extremely vulnerable to a criminal attack.

Condition **CODE YELLOW** is the second level. When you are in condition code yellow you are in relaxed alert and are fully aware of what is around you and you see no specific danger. This is very good.

Condition **CODE ORANGE** is the third level. You sense or see potential danger. Something is not quite right and has your attention. You get mentally prepared to deal with it if necessary. Under condition code orange you may decide to change the course of where you are going and head towards a safer environment.

Condition **CODE RED** is the fourth level and it means imminent danger! When a person is in condition code red someone is attacking them or getting ready to attack them. If you find yourself in condition code red then you most probably will have to defend yourself. In condition code red it is extremely important to react quickly. Pull out your gun, knife, OC pepper spray or other tool of self-defense and be ready to use it. Your life is being threatened. Be ready to fight or run. Usually in condition code red the attacker has gotten too close. Use anything to keep them away from you. Put something between you and them. Yell. Get the attention of others that may be around. Do whatever it takes to survive.

Many attacks involve more than one attacker. Make sure that you keep an eye out for any additional persons that the attacker may have with him or her. Get into the habit of looking for a second person if you have someone unexpectedly approach you. It is a very common tactic to have someone distract the potential victim while another person does the assault.

You need to get into the habit of being aware not just on the street, but also in various other situations such as when someone knocks on your door, when going in or out of your house or car, when traveling, etc.

I remember one time when I went up to a bank kiosk machine to withdraw money. I was facing the street with my back to the parking lot of a grocery store. Fortunately, I am in the habit of taking a good look to make sure that there isn't anyone around that shouldn't be. What I noticed when I looked around was a guy that was about fifty yards away walking across the front sidewalk of the market and initially not in my direction. When I got up to the ATM, I looked into the mirror mounted on it and saw the guy directly behind and walking towards me. I watched him in the mirror until he was about thirty feet behind me. I then turned and told him not to come any closer. He was a big guy and a lot younger than me. He smiled and continued to come towards me. I told him again not to come any closer. I made it clear that I meant what I said by the tone of my voice and my body language. He stopped coming forward. I finished my banking transaction and left.

Let me be clear. Big young guys don't make ninety-degree turns and sneak up on someone getting cash from an instant teller. Who knows what he was up to. Perhaps he just wanted to hustle me for money. Perhaps he wanted to put fear into me so that I would give him money to leave me alone. Or perhaps he had something more sinister in mind. All I know is that I went home safe and with all of my money.

Being aware of potential threats that can exist in any given situation can save you from being a victim.

Protect Yourself from Violence

Avoiding Trouble

The best advice that I have ever heard on this topic is to **"stay away from dangerous places, dangerous situations and dangerous people."** You don't need to increase the risk of something happening to you. Avoiding potential trouble is to reduce the risk of something bad happening to you. Do you really need to go, for example, and hang out at a nightclub known to attract troublemakers where fights break out on a regular basis? Think about what you are doing in your life that increases the possibilities of being in the wrong place at the wrong time. Just because something bad hasn't happened to you so far doesn't mean that something bad can't happen in the future.

Be careful about letting strangers near you. If you don't know someone, it's probably a good idea to not let that person get too close. Also be careful when being nice or helpful to strangers. Criminals are very good at tricking their victims. Whatever you do, don't let someone that you don't know into your home or automobile. If you allow that to occur you have just put yourself at risk of being robbed, assaulted or murdered.

I recently had a person come to the door of my home and try to convince me that I should consider using his services. I felt uncomfortable because he kept coming on too strong. He had a big smile, constantly getting into my personal space and trying to get me to shake his hand. I wouldn't and finally told him that I don't shake hands with someone that I don't know. I could have been nice and shook his hand, but why should I have put myself at risk and allow a stranger that I felt uncomfortable with not only get closer to me, but also have access to a part of my body. He could have been a criminal that held onto my hand and then attacked me (perhaps even used a chemical or electrical device on me). Why should I have taken the chance and put my family at risk?

Keeping your distance from potential threats not only can help you to avoid threats but can also provide you with more time to react to a given threat that you cannot avoid. Adequate reaction time is critical and can save you from being a victim.

To be safe you need to avoid situations that increase your personal risk. Avoid going into dangerous parts of town. Avoid going out late at night. Avoid taking shortcuts where you can't be seen. Avoid crowds – they can turn very quickly from being seemingly safe to being dangerous. Lastly, avoid getting too close to strangers. **Learn to see potential danger before it happens.**

Start looking for the "3-D" things around you and avoid:
- Dangerous places
- Dangerous situations
- Dangerous people

Preparing for Trouble

The best way to survive a violent criminal encounter is to prepare for one before it happens. That way you will have the mindset, the tools, and hopefully the training to defend yourself quickly and efficiently.

It is far better to be prepared before something happens than to learn proper self-defense after you have been victimized. Learning to protect yourself is good. It is much better if you are proactive instead of reactive.

I have met a number of people who have been victims of violence and learned how to better defend themselves afterwards. I know women who have studied martial arts or acquired firearms after being sexually assaulted. I know men who have been mugged and then took measures to protect themselves from future violence.

Whether you have been previously victimized or not, my advice is to learn how you can prepare yourself so that you are hopefully not a victim in the future. This means being mentally tough, being aware of your surroundings, staying away from trouble and being prepared to defend yourself. This means having a survival mentality.

PROTECT YOURSELF FROM VIOLENCE

Your Survival Mentality

Your ability to survive in an increasingly violent world will depend upon your willingness to learn not to be a victim. You will have to pay your dues to do this. This means that you have to spend the time to learn how to see the world differently. You can no longer go through your life in an unaware mental state as to the potential dangers that are around you. You need to learn to look at everything in your life from the point of view of potential danger, how you can avoid these dangers, and how you can defend yourself if you are attacked.

The most important tool that you have for being safe is your mindset. It is what will define your survival mentality. Are you willing to be tough mentally? Are you willing to be disciplined enough to do things differently and keep yourself out of harm's way? Are you willing to be ruthless if attacked? Are you willing to fight dirty? Are you willing to fight to the death if need be to save your family? Have you considered just what you are willing to do to survive a criminal attack?

There is a price that everyone must pay for success. If you want to be a successful bicycle rider you have to spend time learning about and riding your bicycle. If you want to be successful at fishing, then you have to spend time learning how to fish and then spend the needed time fishing. If you want to be good at anything you have to learn about that thing and then put in the time getting good at it. Well the same holds true about learning how to not be a victim. You will have to pay your dues. You will have to make up your mind whether you are willing to do what it takes to be proficient at being safe.

Only you can determine what preparations you need and are willing to do to deter or survive violence. Choose wisely. Your personal safety may depend upon it.

Self-Defense Decisions

Fighting can be bad for you. It is against the law and you should avoid it if you can. Unfortunately, you might not have a choice but to defend yourself. As a rule, you probably need to treat any physical aggression toward you as a criminal assault.

The police and justice system do not look favorably on fighting. So if you can, avoid or talk your way out of getting into one. You don't want to get arrested and possibly spend large amounts of time and money defending yourself in a court of law.

That said you don't want to be a victim either. Being aware and avoiding problems is of course the safest and wisest course of action. But if you are in danger from criminal assault, then you may have no choice but to defend yourself. You have to accept that if you choose to defend yourself you risk being arrested and having to deal with the criminal justice system.

Remember, your goal is not to win a fight. Your goal is to go home intact.

Please, whatever you do, don't lose your temper and do something stupid that makes the criminal appear to be the victim and you the aggressor.

Protect Yourself from Violence

Part II
Tools

Self-Defense Options

There are many self-defense options available. They all have their pros and cons depending on what you are mentally and physically capable of doing. Most are tools and all can help protect you. Some of these tools are weapons (guns and knives for example). Some are things made for other purposes that can be used as weapons (such as golf clubs and baseball bats).

Others are designed to stop an attacker while avoiding or minimizing lethal force (such as pepper spray and stun guns). Still others are devices that can deter a criminal assault under some situations (such as horns and whistles). Lastly, there is the option of defending yourself with just your hands and feet. All of these self-defense options have their strengths and weaknesses. Further in the book I will discuss these options in more detail and what you can realistically expect from each of them.

The main point that I am trying to make is that you should consider all of the self-defense options that are available to you before deciding which one/ones you will use. When considering your options you need to consider the level of potential violence that you may encounter where you live, work and travel. You also need to consider what you are capable of actually being able to use or do. Lastly you will also need to evaluate your possible options in light of what you can legally employ in your self-defense.

Self-defense options can be grouped into the following general categories:

Projectiles: Guns, bows and arrows, throwing knives, blowguns, spears, slingshots, rocks, etc.

Cutting tools: knives, machetes, swords, ice picks, spears, razors, box cutters, axes, tomahawks, hatchets, etc.

Impact: Batons, sticks, pipes, umbrellas, walking sticks and canes, golf clubs, baseball bats, rolled-up magazines and newspapers, chains, belts with heavy belt buckles, whips, Kubotans, metal pens, keys between fingers, etc.

Chemicals: Mace®, pepper spray.

Electrical: Stun guns, Tasers®.

Noise: Whistles, air horns, personal alarms.

Light (*for temporary vision impairment*): Camera flash bulbs, powerful flashlights.

Hands and feet (*assumes ability or training*): Martial arts, boxing, wrestling, brawling, street fighting, etc.

Why You Should Carry a Weapon

Every mentally healthy person should carry at least one weapon or other self-defense tool. And you should carry it with you at all times. No exceptions, unless it is not legal to do so. If attacked by criminals, having a means to deter or stop them is essential to your survival.

It doesn't take long for someone to take the life of another. Don't let it be yours. Even the biggest, toughest, best fighters, martial artists, etc., can be overwhelmed or defeated. Life is not fair and no one is invincible. Be prepared to come home intact. Have at least one weapon or other self-defense tool on you at all times. It is great personal insurance.

When anyone carries a weapon, that person has a tremendous responsibility to be safe and to consider using that weapon only when faced with **imminent and unavoidable great bodily harm/loss of life for themselves or their love ones**. This responsibility is not to be taken lightly. You are not John or Jane Bad Ass. You are John or Jane good citizen and need to never get into a situation that you can avoid or walk safely away from. And you must at all times be in control of your emotions. If you are a hot head and tend to get emotionally worked up, then don't carry a weapon. Period. You could land up being in serious trouble and very sorry that you did.

I would like to point out that when threatened with criminal attack, many citizens have avoided violence by simply displaying their weapon. I am not talking about showing it off to impress someone with how deadly you are or that you would love nothing more than to cause them harm. I am talking about letting them know where things will go if they do not back off at once. It has been estimated that every year guns are used as a deterrent approximately nine out of ten times that they are taken out in self-defense situations without a shot being fired. The same type of deterrence can occur with other weapons such as with your knife.

Remember, most criminals prefer to find an easy victim and usually don't want to risk getting hurt.

I would also like to point out that you risk being charged with brandishing a weapon if you take one out to deter a criminal threat. Make sure that you are truly at risk of **imminent and unavoidable great bodily harm/loss of life for yourself or your love ones** if you do. And if a criminal is not deterred when you then take it out you will be on much firmer legal ground if you are forced to use it.

It is strongly recommended that you do not take out your weapon unless you are mentally prepared to use it. If you take it out as a deterrent and are not prepared to use it then you can be seriously hurt or killed by the attacker if he/she continues with the attack.

Lastly, don't underestimate weapons as **force multipliers**. This means that with the use of weapons a person can more effectively defend themselves against bigger, better trained, armed and multiple opponents. This is the equivalent of leveling the playing field more in your favor.

Guns – The Great Equalizer

Guns are called the great equalizer for a very good reason. For example, an athletic criminal weighing 250 pounds can be easily stopped by a little old lady weighing 95 pounds that is armed with a gun. Without the gun, that same little old lady would probably end up a victim even if armed with another type of weapon such as a knife or a stick.

Even if you are young, strong and trained in self-defense you can be overwhelmed by the sheer number of attackers. This is another situation where having a firearm on you can stop the attackers in their tracks and allow you to go home safely.

Many women carry a firearm to prevent being the victim of a sexual assault. A firearm can easily neutralize the physical strength of any man.

As stated in the previous section, just the sight of a gun usually ends a potentially bad situation because criminals know the damage that one can do.

I am not going to go into great detail about guns. There are literally thousands of different guns that have been manufactured. And there are many good books and videos on the subject as well as many knowledgeable folks at various gun clubs, shooting ranges and stores across the country that can provide you with the specific information that you may need or be seeking.

In this section I will provide a brief overview of firearms and their value for self-protection for the average person.

Basically, guns can be grouped into three distinct groups: handguns, rifles and shotguns. These three types are designed for different purposes but each type can be used very effectively for self-defense depending on the situation that the user may be in.

Handguns

Handguns come in two basic types: the semi-automatic pistol and the revolver. Yes, I know that there are single and double shot derringers and other guns that don't precisely fall into one of the two categories, but most handguns manufactured and purchased are of these types.

The semi-automatic pistol holds a magazine and automatically loads the next round of ammunition (loaded cartridge) into the firing chamber of the gun. They usually hold more rounds of ammunition than the revolver. They also have more moving parts and require more attention than the revolver. The semi-automatic pistol is usually what you see in action movies and its what most police departments and military branches utilize. For those who are willing to get proficient with their firearm, both training and maintenance, then the semi-automatic pistol can be a superior gun because of the capacity of rounds of ammunition in the gun and the speed and ease of changing magazines (and hence having more rounds available). This feature can save your life in some situations. The semi-automatic pistol is the preferred gun for many people for self-defense but requires a

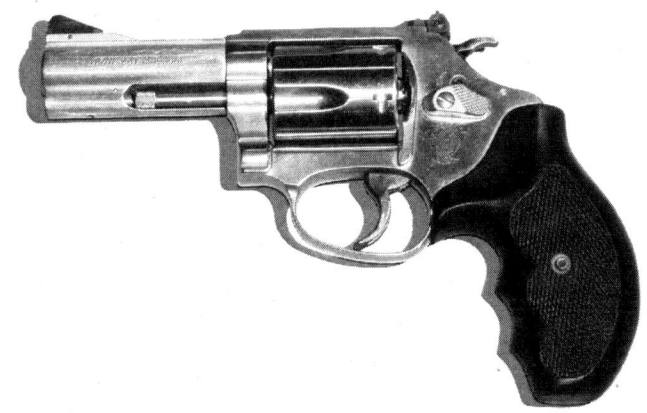

The Smith and Wesson model 60 revolver in .357 caliber also shoots the .38 Special cartridge. Photo courtesy of Ron Kibler and Jered Hallstrom.

bit more training and knowledge to get good with.

The revolver is the gun known as the six-shooter (or wheel gun) although they come in other capacities. These are the guns that you often see in westerns and in the "Dirty Harry" movies. They are less complex than the semi-automatic pistols, but generally hold less rounds of ammunition. The good thing about them is that if a round does not go off when the trigger is pulled, the gun revolves to the next round and you can continue shooting, unlike semi-automatic pistols. I personally feel that the revolver is the best gun for most novices who don't have much experience or interest in guns. For them it will be reliable and easy to maintain.

Handguns are great for self-defense whether in or out of your home when assailants are relatively close to you. Most are easy to handle, easy to draw and easy to fire. I would like to point out that there is a trend towards lighter handguns

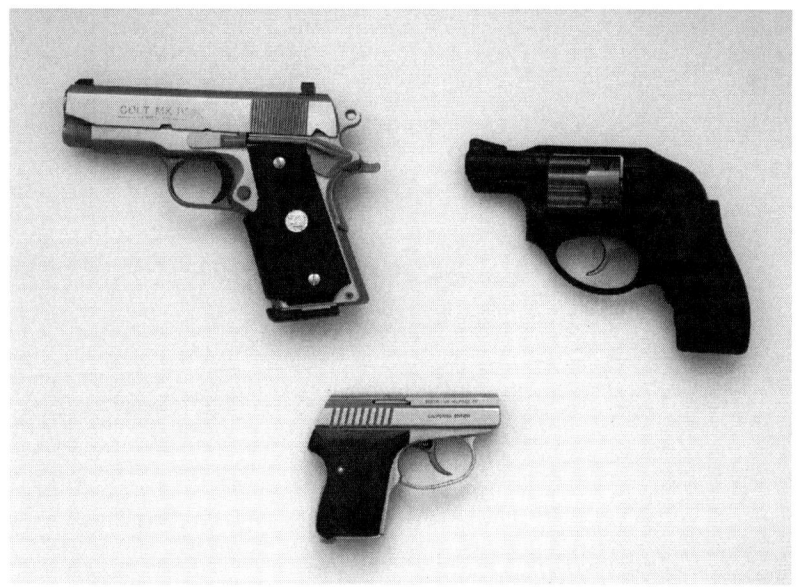

Clockwise from top left: Colt Officer's 45 ACP, Ruger LCP.38 Special Revolver with laser sights and the Seecamp 32 ACP Pistol. The 32 ACP and its small cartridge was the principal caliber carried by police in Europe for decades and can be adequate in many situations. Although it doesn't have optimum stopping power it sure beats not having any firearm when you need to defend yourself.

for personal carry. Some of the guns can be very difficult for many people to shoot well because they are small and light weight. And some have very small cartridges such as .25 or .32 calibers that can make shooting a little easier, but with a loss of stopping power. I know that shot placement can be the difference in stopping someone regardless of caliber, but I recommend that your primary handgun used for self-defense be at least .38 caliber, and preferable larger, because of the increased ability to stop an attacker (in general, the larger the caliber the more damage that it can cause).

Handguns that often hold less ammunition are commonly made lightweight, smaller and hence easier to carry on one's person. I've heard it said that the best handgun to have is the one that you are willing to have on you. Therefore, a small semi-automatic pistol or revolver that you are willing to carry is far superior to a large handgun that you leave at home because of its lack of convenient carry size or weight.

If the felt recoil of a small or lightweight handgun makes it difficult to shoot then you will probably not practice with it very much. But proficiency with a gun is very important because you will do in real life what you practice the most. My recommendation is that you get the smallest gun of adequate caliber that you can shoot well and comfortably as your primary carry handgun. It probably will not be the smallest or the lightest gun made. Also get a good carry holster that is comfortable. You will be willing to carry your gun more if you do so.

Note: as an alternative some people carry an extremely small handgun and own a larger handgun. They do most of their shooting practice with the larger, more manageable handgun. This helps them to maintain a higher level of shooting proficiency while minimizing the discomfort that may come from shooting their smaller handgun. Also, a larger handgun makes an easier to shoot defensive handgun for inside of your home.

Rifles

Rifles come in various sizes, shapes and calibers. They are commonly available in single shot or semi-automatic and they are designed for various purposes. Rifles are made for self-defense, fighting, hunting and target shooting. There are rifles such as the AR-15 that can be used for all the stated purposes. There are rifles such as the bolt action .308 which makes a great hunting and target rifle.

Short barrel rifles, such as carbines, can be very useful for self-defense around the home. Their main benefits are that they can often shoot larger caliber ammunition more comfortably than handguns and that with longer barrels they can offer greater accuracy at distance. Handguns are very quick to maneuver and are reasonably accurate at closer distances, say out to 10 yards. Rifles are not as quick to maneuver but can be very accurate for much greater distances. I would like to point out that the accuracy of any firearm is dependent upon the quality of the gun, its ammunition and the skill of the shooter. I am just trying to provide the reader with some idea of what to expect, in general, with each type of firearm.

Note: for home defense, rifles will give you far greater penetration value, and probably will go through a person and continue to travel through walls. So in most situations, people should consider using handguns and shotguns as their primary self-defense firearms. Rifles, in my opinion, are best if you are defending yourself against attackers that are further away.

GEORGE A. DEFILLIPO

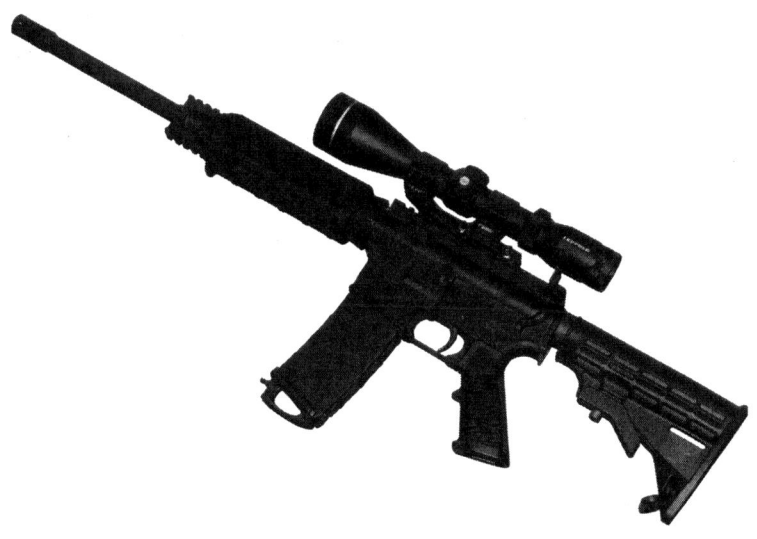

The Smith and Wesson M&P 15 Sport Rifle in .223 caliber.
Contrary to their military looks, AR-15 sporting rifles are
just a variety of semi-automatic firearms.
Photo courtesy of Ron Kibler and Jered Hallstrom.

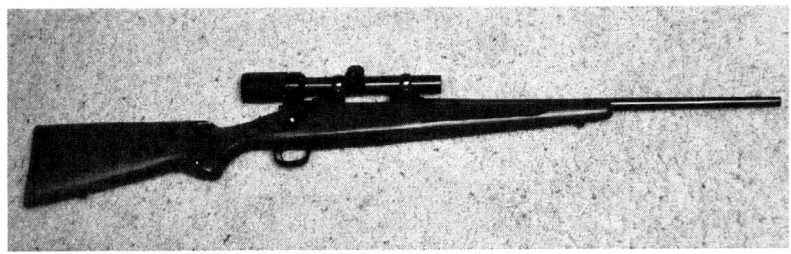

The Winchester Model 70 bolt-action rifle in .223 caliber.
Photo courtesy of Ron Kibler and Jered Hallstrom.

Shotguns

The shotgun (also known as the scattergun) is another thing altogether. It has a large bore and is designed to put out a lot of lead, or other projectiles, in a relatively short distance. There are various designs of shotguns such as pump, semi-automatic, side-by-side, and over-and-under. Each is designed for a different purpose. All can stop a criminal when loaded with the right ammunition. Shotguns made for self-defense most commonly come in pump and semi-automatic with side-by-sides becoming increasingly popular with women. I prefer the pump because of the sound that it makes when loading a shell into the chamber. Just about everyone knows that sound and hearing it often results in the bad guy making a hasty retreat. In addition, pump action shotguns have fewer moving parts than semi-automatic shotguns and are less likely to break down.

A home defense shotgun, usually offered in 12-gauge, will have a shorter barrel than other types of shotguns. This

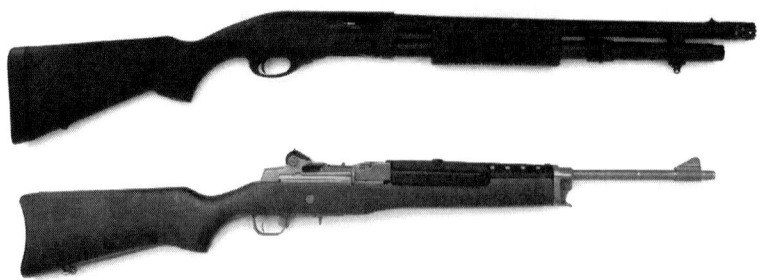

Top: Remington 870 Tactical 12 gauge pump shotgun.
Bottom: Ruger Mini 14 semi-automatic rifle in .223 caliber.

allows for quicker maneuverability. It may also have a long magazine tube for holding more rounds of shotgun shells (usually 4-8). And a home defense shotgun may have the capability to shoot a variety of lengths of shotgun shells that will increase its flexibility as far as ammunition choices are concerned.

There are a lot of opinions regarding which shotgun shells would be best for home defense. Double OO buckshot is very popular. But remember it can easily penetrate dry wall (it can also go through car doors). Some people use smaller shot such as #8 target load for self-defense inside their homes to minimize over penetration and accidental injuries. Remember, at short range, there is a lot of lead or steel coming out of a shotgun with tremendous force regardless of the ammunition type being used.

For most people, a handgun offers the most flexibility in that it can be carried concealed (where legal) and can be available immediately for use in the home. Many people like to have both a handgun and a shotgun for their self-protection.

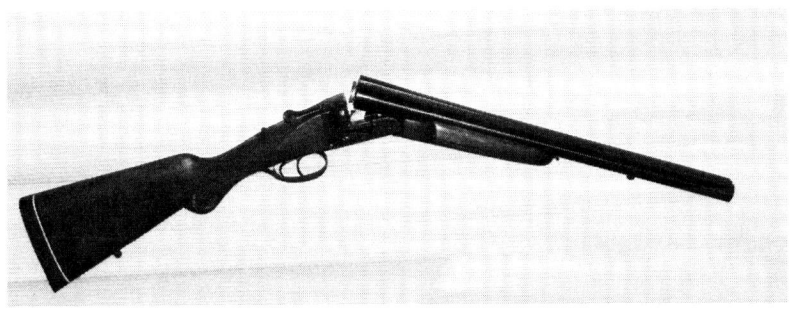

A Spanish Urico 12 gauge side-by-side shotgun.
Photo courtesy of Ron Kibler and Jered Hallstrom.

Note: firearm safety is of paramount importance. Please strictly adhere to the following safe gun handling rules:

- Always assume that every gun is loaded at all times.
- Never point a gun at anything that you are not willing to destroy.
- Keep your finger off the trigger until ready to shoot.
- Always clearly identify your target and what's behind it before shooting.

I recommend that you keep all your firearms locked inside a safe or with trigger locks on them when not being utilized for your security.

If you have a family member with questionable mental stability or anger issues, having your weapon or weapons secured at all times is absolutely necessary both for their safety as well as for the safety of others.

Learn and comply with the firearm laws for where you live.

George A. DeFillipo

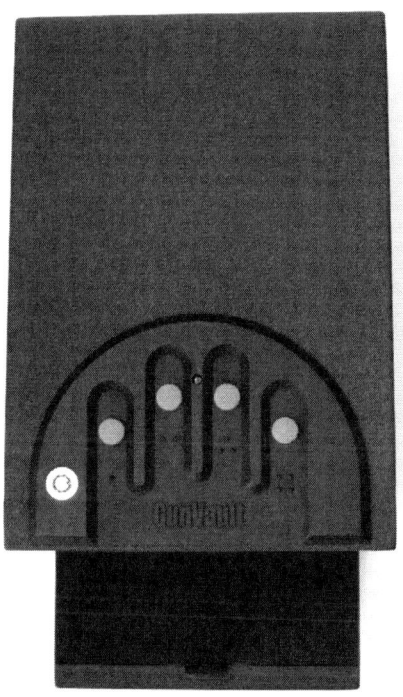

Small handgun safes such as this one from Gun Vault are affordable for most people and keep your weapon out of the hands of those that should not have access to it. In addition, a small handgun safe is easy to hide inside a cabinet or under a bed.

PROTECT YOURSELF FROM VIOLENCE

Knives — When You Don't Have a Gun

Most people don't realize or underestimate what a viable tool for self-defense a knife can be. Since knives are extremely available, it makes sense that they be utilized as tools for personal protection and self-defense.

This section provides information that the average person needs to know about utilizing knives as tools for personal protection. It will briefly explain the differences between basic knife designs used for survival, fighting and self-defense. Fundamental knowledge of knife encounters and street survival will also be covered.

It is also the purpose of this section to explain the pros and cons of the basic concepts of self-defense with a bladed weapon within the context of modern society. There will be no attempt to teach the reader knife self-defense techniques. This book is not a replacement for professional instruction in knife usage. Those who desire to become proficient in this area need to seek out a reputable source of training.

Knives have their place although guns are the preferred weapons for personal protection and self-defense in most situations. Quality knives never malfunction or run out of ammunition and may be all that you can legally carry now or in the future.

Section I

Knife Design for Personal Protection

Knives for Human Encounters Made For Other Purposes

Knives come in all sizes and shapes and are made for many purposes such as kitchen knives, hunting and fishing knives, skinning knives, general utility knives, combat and tactical knives, and survival knives to name some of the most common. All can cut and most can stab. The purpose of stating this is that you most probably already have knives that can work in a pinch to defend yourself and your loved ones if the need was to arise. If you are at home, they are probably accessible to you at the moment. You are not necessarily weaponless if you don't own a knife designed for self-defense. Just look in your kitchen and other places around your home or garage.

The Survival Knife and the Fighting Knife

There are knives that by their design are superior for personal protection and self-defense. They include some survival knives (if well made), fighting and combat knives, many tactical knives, and a number of personal folder knives. Some hunting knives can have many of the attributes

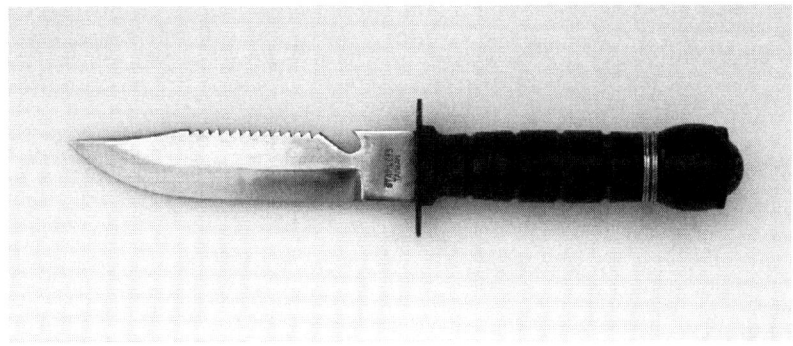

Cheap imported survival knife – stay away from them as they cannot be trusted to hold-up without breaking.

of fighting knives; make sure they have those that you are looking for, especially length.

The survival knife can be used as a fighting knife. It is primarily designed for work and uses other than fighting. It can have a hollow handle for holding survival items such as a whistle, fish hooks, fishing line, compass, etc. Many survival knives available are cheaply made and are not going to hold up to heavy use and can break at the wrong time. There are some well-made survival knives that you can depend on, but they will require more sharpening and other maintenance when used primarily as a work knife. If you can find one that is made with quality components and you are prepared to keep it razor sharp, then this choice is a viable option. Many quality survival knives do not have hollow handles, but rather their handles are shaped for optimal grip and comfort. Survival knives are usually heavier than fighting knives because they are designed for various work tasks such as the chopping that is needed to construct a temporary structure from tree limbs in the wilderness.

Even with the design emphasis of doing work over fighting, a quality survival knife can be a very good knife for personal protection for most people. It can have many of the qualities of a fighting knife and can be extremely rugged when constructed with quality components.

Tactical knives originally were military knives modified to accommodate a second useful purpose in addition to

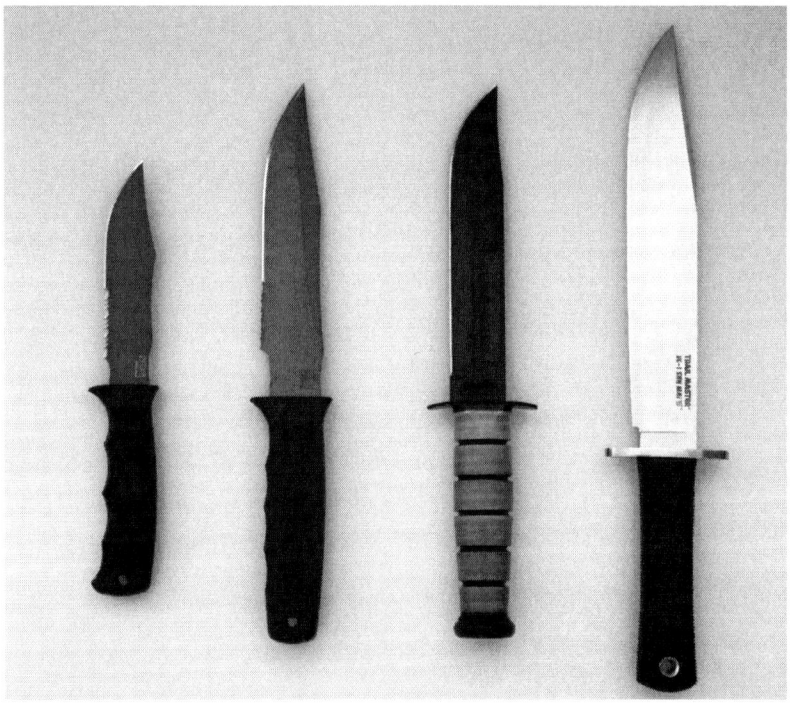

Various quality fixed blade knives from left to right: SOG Navy Seal Pup, SOG Navy Seal, USMC K-Bar and the Cold Steel Trailmaster SAN MAI III. The first three knives can be utilized as combat fighting knives. The Cold Steel Trailmaster SAN MAI III is an all around field knife that can serve as a hunting, survival and fighting knife.

fighting. Over time many of them have become very specialized in their designs to accommodate very specific tactical situations. Currently, there are many designs of tactical knives available on the market. Make sure that if you choose a tactical knife for your protection, it has the design and all the features you need to effectively defend yourself.

There are many fighting knives out there. Some are custom made that cost more than factory manufacture knives. If money is not an issue and you desire owning a custom knife, then by all means buy one. For most people the main thing to consider is spending an adequate amount of money to buy a quality knife from a reputable company. There is nothing worse than buying a cheap knife only to have it break while you are trying to defend yourself. Cheap knives sometimes are not made with metal that goes all the way from the tip of the blade to the end of the handle. Quality knives are. There are many quality knives that are reasonably priced and will do an excellent job of holding up. Examples of manufacturers I am familiar with that make quality knives suitable for self-defense are Benchmade, Buck, Cold Steel, CRKT, Gerber, Ka-Bar, Kershaw, Ontario, SOG, Spyderco and Strider.

Most dedicated fighting knives were developed for fighting (for example the Bowie) or military combat use (for example the Ka-Bar). They are big, usually well made and effective for cutting and/or stabbing. Are you going to be carrying one around with you all the time? My guess is probably not. If you do carry one openly in many places in our society, people will view you as a person carrying a deadly weapon. Carrying a large knife concealed where legal is definitely a viable option. Check your state and local laws before doing so.

If you know ahead of time that you will need a fighting knife, then why wouldn't you just bring a gun or even better yet avoid the situation altogether?

Don't get me wrong. If someone broke into my house and I didn't have quick access to a shotgun or other firearm, then I would surely like to have a well-made fighting knife to defend myself with.

Benefits of a Knife Guard

If I have a choice between two similar high quality fixed blade knives that do everything I need them to do and one has a guard and the other doesn't, I will pick the one with the guard. A guard is a piece of metal extending out from the area between the handle and the blade which helps prevent your hand from making accidental contact with the blade and getting cut. It also helps protect your hand from being cut by an attacker

The Personal Carry Knife

The best knife for self-defense is the one that you are willing to carry or have readily available. For many people this knife is the folder. The folder is popular because it is convenient to carry, fast to access, and it's easy to find one that is legal. Unfortunately, for most people, folders are a hit-and-miss proposition as far as quality and design are concerned.

There are six areas that I look at when evaluating a folder

for purchase (note: the first three listed apply to fixed blade knives also). They are:
1. Quality of the blade (both strength and ability to hold a sharp edge).
2. Design and shape of the blade.
3. Comfort, toughness and grip-ability of the handle.
4. Strength of the locking mechanism.
5. Ease of opening.
6. Pocket clip location and design

Let's look at each of these parts of the folding knife in turn.

Blade Quality

First is the quality of the blade. All blades are not made the same. To produce a knife that can hold up to impact, the blade must not be too brittle. For a blade to hold a really sharp edge it must have characteristics that could make it too brittle if care is not taken in its manufacture. Quality knife manufacturers carefully construct their blades with high quality materials. They use special steels and other metals often combined with various other elements that are carefully processed together resulting in blades that mitigate the problems, producing a sharp cutting edge and resistance to breakage. These fine blades don't come cheap, but through modern manufacturing processes the knives produced with these blades are made affordable. In my opinion, spending a little more for a knife with a quality blade is money well spent. Besides, how much is your life worth?

Examples of quality steels used in self-defense and fighting knife blades that I am familiar with include carbon steels: 1040, 1045, 1050, 1055, 1060, 1080, 1085, 1095, SK-5, and stainless steels such as: 9CRV19MOV, 154CM, 420HC, ATS 34, AUS 8, AUS 8A, CPM S30V, D-2, VG-1, and VG-10. Damascus steel makes for an incredible blade if made properly, but is expensive.

Note: There are knives being produced with laminated construction, such as the SAN MAI III (a registered trademark of Cold Steel, Inc.), that sandwich harder steel between layers of softer steel. The stated benefits of this design are that the harder steel will provide a very sharp edge that is longer lasting and the tough outer steel layers will provide increased resistance to breakage.

Blade Design and Shape

Second is the blade design and shape. Are you looking for a knife primarily for stabbing? Then a narrow straight blade with a sharp point is probably what you are looking for such as the dagger. If cutting and slashing is your primary style of self-defense, then you might want a curved blade design such as the Ghurka's Kukri knife that is capable of incredible amounts of cutting, but stabbing is minimized and can be awkward. Or lastly, do you want a blade that can do a good job stabbing and cutting, an all-around versatile knife, but not quite as effective at cutting or stabbing as the specialized cutting or stabbing knives mentioned above?

Some people prefer a knife with a partially serrated blade and others not. A serrated blade gives you increased blade

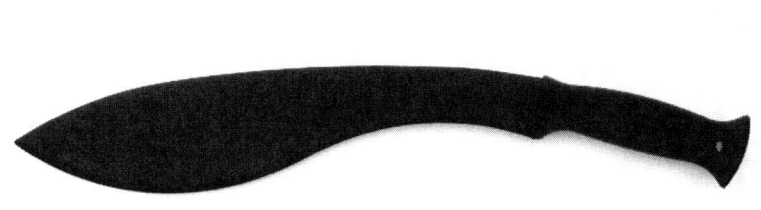

Kurki machete made by Cold Steel

cutting surface, but is more difficult to keep sharpened. If you use your knife for everyday cutting chores and are willing and able to keep it razor sharp, then a serrated blade can be a viable choice for you. If you find sharpening a serrated blade to be too difficult, then I recommend a straight blade because of its ease of sharpening. If you do not use your blade for everyday use, then owning a serrated blade is just fine because it is always ready in a razor sharp state.

Handle Design, Toughness and Grip-Ability

Third is the handle design and the material that it is made of. Does the handle fit your hand comfortably? Could it slip out of your grip when wet, such as if you are forced to defend yourself in the rain or if it gets covered in blood? Find out what the handle material is made of and make sure it has the grip-ability that you need. Also, make sure that the handle material is tough and won't break or come loose in a self-defense situation.

Locking Mechanism

Fourth is the design and strength of the locking mechanism. When I evaluate the locking mechanism I try to determine if the blade will always securely lock into position when the blade is fully extended. I also look to see if the locking mechanism is sturdy and uncomplicated. Simple and strong are good. This is more important than most people realize. The last thing you will want to happen in an altercation while using your folding knife is to have the locking mechanism fail and your fingers severely cut. Defending yourself with a folding knife that doesn't have a locking mechanism can have similar disastrous results.

Ease of Opening

Fifth is the ease of opening the knife. Where legally permitted, you should be able to open any folder knife used for personal protection with one hand. It should not require any special manipulation or extra movement on your part. Initiating the opening should be easy and require minimal effort. Once the opening process is started, it should open completely, smoothly and quickly. If you have difficulty opening it when not under the stress of being attacked, then how can you depend on being able to open it when your life is on the line?

Note: some personal protection folding knives may be easily opened by others and not by you. Everyone is different. Seek a knife that you are comfortable opening. This is critical.

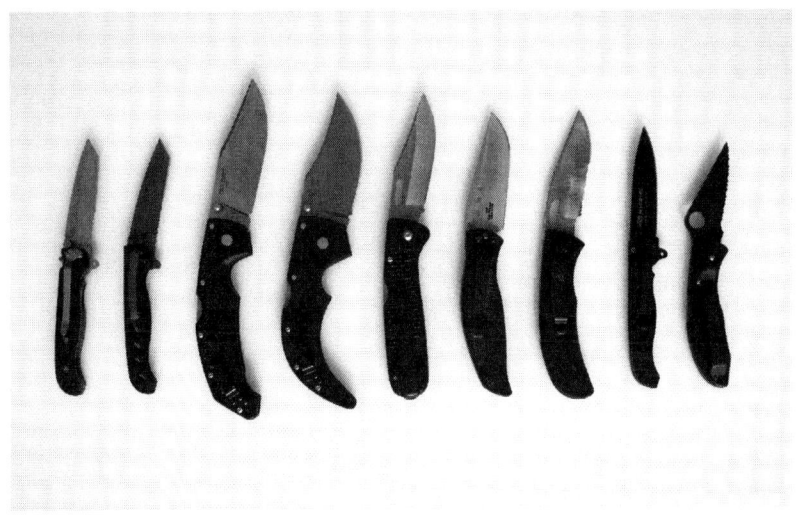

Various folding/pocket knives from left to right: CRKT M16 Tanto, Gerber Tanto, Cold Steel Voyager, Cold Steel Espada, SOG Auto Clip, Kershaw 1560 by Ken Onion, Gerber EZ Out, CRKT M16, and Spyderco Delica

Carry Clip

Sixth is the carry or attachment clip. Your knife should be attached to your pocket or some other location that is easily accessible for quick withdrawal and opening. If you have to turn the knife around before opening it because of the clip's location on the knife, then either you need to relocate the clip or think about choosing a different knife.

Special Caution: due to the large number of counterfeit knives being sold I strongly recommend that you purchase your self-defense knives directly from a manufacturer or an authorized dealer.

Knife Blade Length and Self-Defense

There are advantages and disadvantages that are unique to both long and short blade knives for self-defense. The two most important attributes to be aware of are *reach* and *speed*.

The following sections will provide the reader with the specific pros and cons of each of these two blade length types, including reach and speed.

Long Blade Attributes

The biggest advantage of a knife with a longer blade is *reach*. With a longer blade knife you can keep an attacker farther away from you. You can also strike them, if they have a shorter weapon, before they can strike you. This attribute is huge and can often make the difference between surviving and being a victim of an attack. In addition, if your long blade knife has a forward facing sharp point, then it can better pierce an attacker's body and more easily reach their internal organs for the immediate ending of the attack. If your knife has a sharp edge and a long blade, it will also have the ability to cut deeper and longer because of its extended contact surface and additional weight. Lastly, longer blade knives provide increased leverage and velocity (at the tip), hit harder and therefore have an increased ability to cut and chop. This is a nice attribute to have in a weapon when your life is on the line. A long blade knife may not have the ability to chop off someone's head or limb, but a chop from one can do serious enough damage to immediately end the attack.

In spite of some outstanding attributes of a long blade knife, there are some factors that must be considered if you plan to utilize or carry one. First, because of their size they can be slower to get into action. Second, it can be more difficult to maneuver them in close quarters. Third, they can be more difficult to carry concealed. Fourth, it may be illegal to carry one (openly or concealed) where you live. Still for around the house or out in the back woods, a long blade weapon can be an outstanding self-defense tool to have and well worth owning.

Short Blade Attributes

Short blade knives like smaller guns are more comfortable and easier to carry. Like guns, knives are useless if you do not have one when you need one. And most people are more likely to carry a knife as a self-defense tool if it is easy and comfortable to do so. In addition, short blade knives are legal to carry in more states and cities than longer ones (please check your state and local laws before carrying a knife).

Short blade knives are usually faster to get into action and can be extremely quick in actual self-defense situations. Speed, like reach, is an attribute that can save your life. In addition, unlike long blade knives, short blade knives are ideal for close range because they are much more able to be maneuvered in tight quarters and close contact situations.

The disadvantages of short blade knives are that they do not have the reach or chopping power of longer blade knives. You must engage the attacker when he or she is closer. They

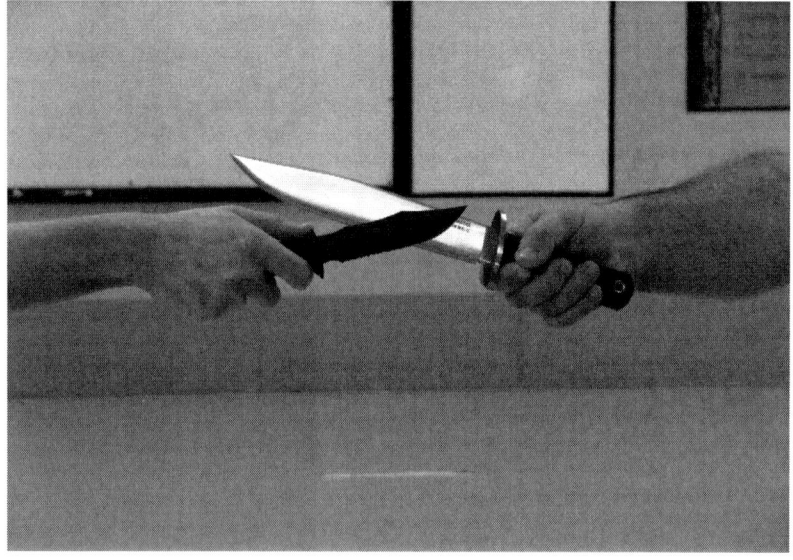

The reach advantage of the longer knife is clearly shown in this photograph.

are not able to penetrate as deeply into the body of an attacker and do not have as much ability to immediately stop them. Lastly, there can be a reduction in cutting capacity.

In spite of these limitations, there are a lot of benefits to carrying a short blade knife. Some knife practitioners carry both long and short blade knives. In my opinion, everyone should at least carry a folder or other small knife with them at all times, where legal.

George A. DeFillipo

Section II

Basic Concepts of Knife Defense

Knife Fighting is Brutal

"Surviving Edged Weapons," the 85-minute police training video from Calibre Press Inc., should be watched by anyone thinking about carrying a knife for self-defense. It is full of re-enactments of crimes committed with knives, some involving police officers. There are photos of real bodies of people that have been killed by knives. These photos are gory. The video shows just how brutal and deadly knives can be. If you think that it is macho to get into a knife fight then think again. The chances of coming out unharmed are not very good. Avoid getting into a knife fight if you can, but if you can't then fight with everything that you have for your life.

There are no absolute guarantees that things will go right with any type of self-defense, but this seems to be especially true when knives are involved. Please make up your own mind as to what you think would work for you. The ideas and concepts presented here are designed to help you survive.

I also would like to strongly recommend that martial artists, proficient in the dojo with various techniques against the knife, only attempt them in real world situations when there are no other options. Trying to keep your distance should always be your first option when possible. It is false bravado to immediately engage someone with a knife if you don't need to and it could get you hurt or killed.

Types of Knife Attacks

There are three types of knife attacks with many variations of each. They are stabbing, slashing and chopping.

Stabbing has been perfected in the prison systems. It is the best means for killing someone behind bars because knives are not available, but stabbing instruments can be made from most anything hard. The typical technique for stabbing, using the ice pick grip, is called "stitching" or "the sewing machine." It usually involves attacking someone from behind with multiple, rapid downward stabs. The target is usually the neck, back and shoulders. The victim can bleed out very quickly.

Another variation of the "stitching" technique developed in prisons involves a frontal approach. The attacker typically has a stabbing weapon in one hand as he approaches the intended victim. When he gets close, he strikes out with his empty hand while frontal stabbing with his other. If things go right for the attacker, the victim can be partially turned away from the attacker and receive numerous stabbing wounds to his abdomen, chest and side. Again, the victim can bleed out very quickly.

Slashing can be done with most any knife, but curved blades, heavier knives and longer length knives are most efficient. A person can be slashed anywhere, but favorite targets include the neck, stomach, legs and arms. Slashing can result in the victim bleeding out very quickly, especially if an artery is severed, leading to unconsciousness and death.

Chopping is the third type of attack that someone with a knife can do. This usually involves using a larger and heavier knife for more serious damage. Many people are killed every year in third world countries from chops delivered by machetes. Don't underestimate chopping in a life or death situation.

Empty Hands Defense Against Stabs, Chops and Slashes

Unless you have formal training and have sufficient practice time doing them, don't attempt to do martial arts techniques against a knife attack. Usually getting away from the attacker or putting something between you and the attacker is your best bet until you can get away. Martial arts techniques exist for overhead stabs and chops, as well as frontal stabs that work quite well. The techniques are with risk even if you have received expert training.

Defense against slashes is much more difficult. Plan on getting cut if you try to disarm a person trying to cut you by slashing. Again, your best bet is to get away or put something between you and the attacker. If you can get to something that you can use as an impact weapon, then you can attempt to strike the attacker's hand.

Note: If you are able to grab the attacker's knife hand and if you are strong enough you can prevent him from stabbing or cutting you. This is not easily done, but if accomplished, can give you the opportunity to wrestle the knife away from the attacker.

Knife Against Knife Defenses

Things can get complicated and very risky when both the attacker and defender have knives. Sometimes just displaying your knife will be enough to convince the attacker that it would not be wise to try something against you, especially if you look determined.

I strongly recommend keeping your distance and using your knife to strike at any part of the attacker's body that he or she extends toward you such as the hands or feet, but especially the hand holding the knife. Do this until you can get away or are forced to use deadly force to defend yourself. Again, don't let the attacker get close to you if you can avoid it. Close quarter knife fighting can be extremely damaging to you. Be ready to move. And as previously stated, put objects between you and the attacker such as vehicles, furniture, etc. so that he or she cannot reach you.

Knife Defense Against Impact Weapons

By impact weapons I mean sticks, clubs, batons, pipes, etc. Impact weapons are usually longer than most knives and therefore have the reach advantage. The reach advantage can be huge and can put the attacker at a serious disadvantage. I personally would rather fight a person that has a knife if I have the impact weapon. So please, stay away from anything that can be used as an impact weapons.

If you must go up against a person who has an impact weapon, try to wait (if you can) until after they make a move and before they can reset before you try to counter and cut

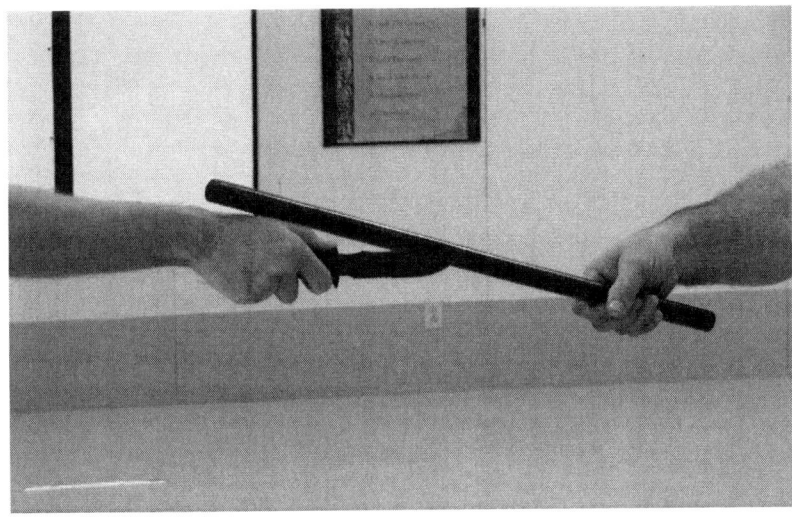

Even though the person on the left has a knife, the reach advantage clearly goes to the person holding the stick.

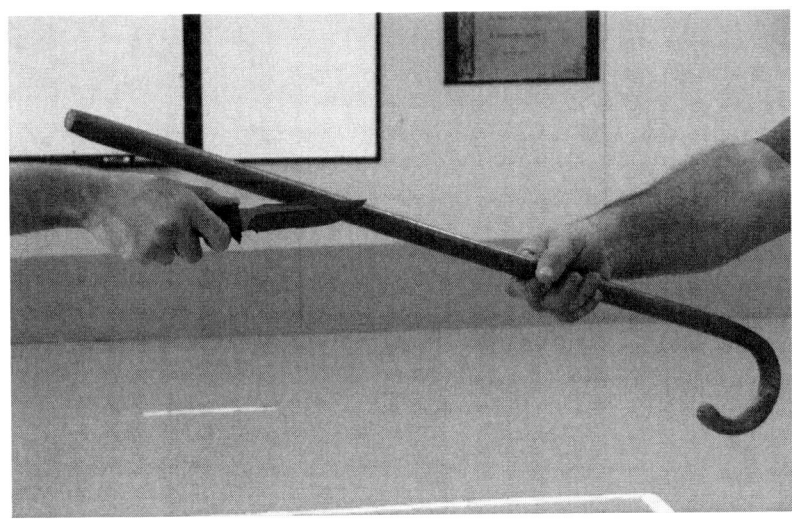

A cane can be an excellent tool for self-defense in many situations. Note: it also has the reach advantage against the knife in this photograph.

them. The hand, wrist and forearm of the weapon hand are excellent targets. This also is very risky to carry out. Again, seek professional training to get proficient in this area.

Improvised Knives

If you don't have a gun or knife and you do have access to objects around you that can be used as or made into knives, then you can still defend yourself. Scissors, pens, pencils, knitting needles, ice picks, screwdrivers etc. can make great-improvised knives for stabbing. In addition, knives can be made from sharp objects such as broken glass from a bottle top. All of these can be used to successfully stop an attacker.

Other Weapons For Use Against Knives

Getting away from an attacker is usually your best bet. If you cannot get away then deterring the attacker by displaying the kind of force that you are capable of using can be your next most viable option.

If getting away or deterring the attacker are not possible solutions at that moment then you will have to use some type of effective force. Effective force is the force that will stop an attacker from hurting you. Tools and weapons that can provide effective force include guns, impact weapons and knives. They are effective because they are all **force multipliers** capable of neutralizing the attacker's force.

Guns provide the most immediate stopping power of

any self-defense tools in most situations. Guns provide the best means of stopping an attacker with the least amount of risk of injury to yourself. After these I find impact weapons to be great tools for self-defense against the knife. OC pepper spray can buy you some time to get away from your attacker.

By the way, if someone is close to you and attacking with a knife and you have a gun, don't hesitate to use it. The damage that a person with a knife can do to you if you don't stop them can be enormous. They are using deadly force against you. If you are unclear on this matter, then re-watch the video "Surviving Edged Weapons" or watch the news video from Chontales, Nicaragua showing a man attacking multiple police officers with a large knife. He killed two of them and wounded others even though the officers were armed with AK 47 rifles. You can find this video by typing the following on your computer: November 2010 knife attack Chontales, Nicaragua.

Section III

Surviving Real Life Encounters with a Knife

"When speaking of survival, we're not talking about two individuals who choose to fight each other; we are talking about being attacked. Most attacks are unexpected, brutal and over quickly. We want to prepare our students to survive such realistic situations." (From the American Practical Arnis Student Handbook.)

Being Prepared

Having a survival mindset is key. It means being mentally and physically prepared for a very dangerous and unpredictable world. To be prepared you need to always be armed. If you don't have a knife or other weapon with you, then how can you use it to defend yourself? It also means that your knife is kept *razor sharp* at all times and that you have it with you at all times. It means that you have your knife where it is easily accessible and that you have sufficient practice taking it out quickly. Lastly, it means being willing to use your knife to defend yourself or as a deterrent.

The Knife as a Deterrent

Criminals will often leave a potential victim alone if it is believed that he or she is armed. They will just seek out easier prey. It is estimated that guns are used as a deterrent in nine out of ten situations without having to fire them. Just taking them out is enough. Knives can do the same thing. I have personally observed this to be true and so have many other people. Remember, you can be accused of brandishing a weapon if you do so.

I believe that many criminals will avoid attacking a person armed with a knife, even a folding knife, if it is easily seen and the person displays a mind-set that they are not to be messed with.

If You Have to Defend Yourself With a Knife

Whatever you do, don't take the fight to the ground unless you are sure that you are fighting just one attacker.

Make it clear to any witnesses that you are the victim. Yell for help or for the police. Be loud. Get public attention.

After the fight call the police immediately if it is safe to do so. Be very careful what you say to the 911 dispatch operator. What you say can be used against you in a court of law. Sometimes the criminal will call the police first and claim to be the victim. It is not unusual for the police to treat the first person to call them as the victim. If this occurs, then you could be treated as the one who did the attacking.

If it is not safe to stay at the site of the attack (like when the attacker's friends are around), then I recommend that you consider leaving immediately and call the police as soon as you are in a safe location. Explain to the police that you left because of fear for your safety. Be very careful what you say during this 911 call. Remember, you can be accused of leaving the scene of a crime if you do.

If you are injured, go to a hospital immediately, even if the wound seems minor. Ask the hospital staff to call the police and state that you were a victim of an attack.

Summing-up the Main Pros and Cons of Utilizing Knives for Self-Defense

There are many benefits to utilizing knives for self-defense. These include:
- Readily available.
- Affordable.
- Can be an excellent deterrent to criminals.
- Can be convenient to carry.
- Formidable weapons, especially with training.
- They are force multipliers.

There are some potential negatives to utilizing knives for self-defense. These include:
- Defense must be at close range.
- Less immediate stopping power than firearms.
- May be illegal to own or carry where you live.

The Power of Impact Weapons

In the right situation impact weapons can be fantastic tools for ending a violent attack. Striking someone with a stick or cane is a viable means of self-defense. Striking someone with a baseball bat or golf club likewise will do the job.

If you decide to use an impact weapon to defend yourself, remember that you must strike your attacker decisively. If you do not really apply enough power to your strike, then you probably will just have a pissed-off attacker on your hands that will want to rip your head off. Make sure that you have ample room to really swing or thrust with your impact weapon. And put your body into it, especially your hips.

Remember, you must strike the person with enough force to stop them cold. If you hit someone with wimpy strikes, you will probably not get the job done. If you are not sure as to how much power to use, then get the opinion of someone who can watch you swing your impact weapon. If you respect that person's judgment and they say it *should* do the job, then continue to work at it until you make it even more powerful. If they say it *will* do the job then you probably have an effectively powerful swing or thrust. Remember to use more power, not less, as you practice.

Great targets for impact weapons are the hands, feet, knees and head.

Remember, you can be accused of using deadly force if you choose to use an impact weapon for your self-defense. So make sure that you are using it only when faced with **imminent and unavoidable great bodily harm/loss of life for yourself or a love one.**

Other Tools for Self-Defense

There are many items out there that can be used for your self-defense besides what have been listed in the previous three chapters. Some are weapons. Others are tools and devices designed to deter. And others still are made for an entirely different purpose, but can be used for self-defense. I recommend staying with guns, knives and impact-weapons as your primary self-defense tools, but you may desire utilizing some of these other choices to enhance your security.

Mace® and pepper spray are chemical deterrents. They are known to work on most people if they are breathed in or get into the eyes. Unfortunately, they are not foolproof. Some people, such as persons on drugs, don't seem to be as affected by them as others. In addition you need to get the spray out in a hurry and spray it accurately on the attacker. It is not always easy to do under the stress of a violent encounter. Overall, if the person being attacked is prepared and uses Mace® or pepper spray at the moment of attack, it can give him/her the time needed to escape in many situations.

Where legal, Tasers® and stun guns can work well in very specific situations. They are considered non-lethal tools that can be used to stop an attacker or used as a deterrent. Both devices use high voltage with low amperage electricity. Tasers® shoot electrical probes with wires through the air

PROTECT YOURSELF FROM VIOLENCE

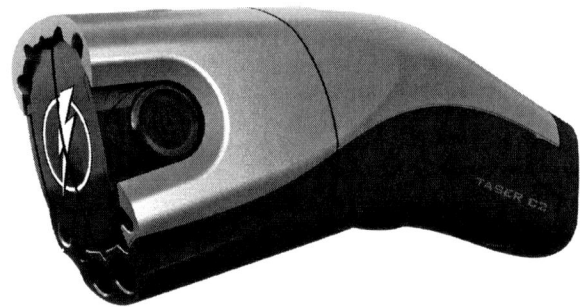

Taser ® C2 ™ is a top of the line product with the highest take down power. It can be used up to a 15 foot distance and comes with an integrated laser sight and holster. Photo courtesy of Dana Leigh Shafman, Shieldher, Inc. For more information or to purchase this product please contact www.shieldher.com or call 602-881-0802. Mention code: PYFV.

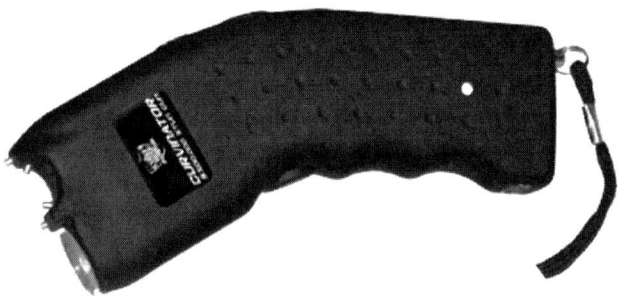

Curvinator 9.5 stun gun is powerful with 9,500,000 volts. Photo courtesy of Streetwise Security Products, streetwisesecurity.net. For more information or to purchase the 9.5 Curvinator Stun Gun, please contact: Howard Whitman, Centerpoint Security Products, 951-551-1249 or shopcsp@gmail.com. Mention code: PYFV

onto the targeted person that results in involuntary submission through neuromuscular incapacitation. This can be done at a safe distance and can give you up to 30 seconds to get to safety before the attacker can move. The stun gun requires the user to hold the electrical probes against that person and utilizes pain to stop the attacker. Once the stun gun is turned-off the attacker is able to move once again. Many law enforcement agencies find Tasers® and stun guns to be very effective tools.

Caution: although stun guns and Tasers® are considered non-lethal, they can still injure a person or animal. Only use when necessary for your self-defense.

Bright flashlights and camera flashbulbs work very nicely to temporarily blind an attacker and flashlights can also be utilized as impact weapons.

Kubotans are tools frequently used by police and martial artists and are also available to citizens for purchase. They are hand-held small cylinder shaped tools designed to provide compliance by inflicting immediate controlled pain. They can also be used as impact weapons. Training in the use of these tools is highly recommended and can be found at many martial arts studios.

Whistles, air horns and personal alarms are deterrents. They can work quite well in well-populated situations, especially air horns and loud personal alarms, as most criminals do not like to be noticed. Unfortunately, they are probably of little help if there aren't a lot of people around.

Improvised weapons can save your life. An example of an improvised weapon is the common pen (or pencil). It can be used very effectively for stabbing, especially to soft tissue such as the neck and eyes. Another example would

PROTECT YOURSELF FROM VIOLENCE

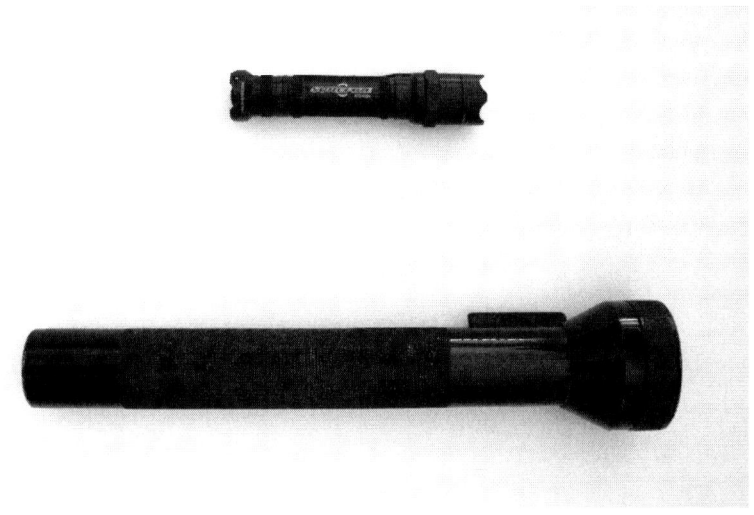

Tactical flashlights can temporarily blind and provide the time
to escape or be used for self-defense as an impact weapon.
Top: Surefire E2D Executive Defender.
Bottom: Streamlight SL-20.

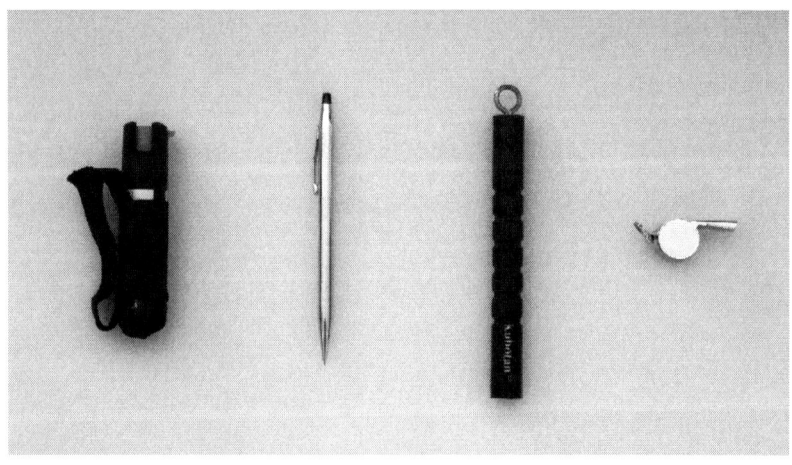

Tools that can be used to defend yourself with from left to right: OC
pepper spray, metal mechanical pencil, Kubotan with key holder,
and a whistle for attracting attention.

be holding your keys so that they stick out between your fingers. A strike with keys can result in the attacker receiving serious pain.

PROTECT YOURSELF FROM VIOLENCE

Martial Arts, Boxing, Wrestling And Other Self-Defense Hand-To-Hand Fighting Systems

Learning a self-defense system has many benefits for anyone willing to put in the time and is physically able to do the various movements involved. It generally takes years of dedicated effort to get proficient enough to be able to defend yourself against a street tough person with just your hands and feet.

When a person learns a self-defense system, they go through various stages of development, learning simple moves to those more complex. With enough repetition of those moves they become increasingly automatic reflexes that your body just performs when presented with the given stimulus. Obviously, a person with extensive self-defense training has an advantage over someone without this training, all things being equal. I have personally seen some highly trained individuals do some incredible things.

Nowadays we are bombarded by an endless supply of movies where the stars (or their stunt doubles) win fights against seemingly overwhelming odds. It makes for great entertainment. Unfortunately, the reality is that most of the fight scenes in these movies have to be filmed numerous times in spite of the carefully planned choreography, because they are so difficult to execute precisely. In the real world many of the fight scenes seen in these movies just wouldn't work.

The truth is self-defense systems can make a person better able to defend himself/herself, but there are limitations. I am not going into these in great detail except to state that learning a self-defense system doesn't make someone invincible. If there are too many opponents, especially if they are armed, or bigger or tougher, then good luck thinking that you will walk away unscathed just armed with your fighting skills.

Another thing to think about is what techniques will be most effective on the street in real encounters, especially when you get older. This is what you should focus your energies on, rather than fancy moves that work nicely only in the ring or on the mat.

There are self-defense systems that focus on hitting, kicking, throwing, locking joints, grappling, using weapons, or some combination of these. If you are interested in learning a self-defense system, it would be prudent to observe some classes from different systems to see which would best work with your body type, age, natural inclination, etc. I recommend finding a system that has been around for a while and has proven its effectiveness over time. Lastly, when you find a self-defense system that matches your needs, make sure that you find an instructor of that system who is good at teaching and fighting.

I would like to point out that it is fine to learn how to defend yourself on the ground if the fight ends up there. But I will caution you to not take any fight to the ground if you can avoid it, even if you believe that you are fighting only one person. It increases your vulnerability to possible unforeseen factors such as the arrival of additional attackers.

Overall, learning a self-defense system will make you better fit physically and increase your self-confidence. You will be better able to defend yourself and will be able to react more quickly to whatever situation is at hand. I recommend learning one if you are interested in doing so, as long as you are realistic about the limits associated with this type of self-defense.

Lastly, I strongly recommend that you consider learning how to defend yourself with a weapon such as a knife, stick, etc. This training can greatly improve your chances of going home intact when dealing with street-tough criminals.

Protect Yourself from Violence

Part III
Preparations

The Value of Training

Formal Training

We live in an era where it is common practice for people to take education classes and self-help courses in order to get a better job. Many people likewise enjoy learning about a new hobby or recreational activity and have no problem with spending the time needed to do so. Unfortunately, when it comes to being safe very few people will spend the time and energy learning how to be so. Perhaps it is because many people have lived during times that have been relatively safe in the past. Perhaps it is because it is difficult for people to think about the possibility of something bad happening. Nevertheless, if you want to be safe, then you need to learn the skills associated with doing so.

For example, if you decide to acquire a gun for self-protection, then you will need to learn how to safely and efficiently handle that gun. This includes how to load, aim and fire it. This takes sufficient repetition to be able to do automatically, especially under duress. Many people take classes from accredited firearms instructors or other highly trained persons so that what they learn is learned correctly.

The same holds true for learning any other skill that can help you to be safe such as using pepper spray, a Taser®, a knife, a stick, or even having a well-trained dog at home for self protection. In a real life situation you will do what you have practiced sufficiently. You will most likely not have the time to think about how to properly hold and use your gun, knife, pepper spray, Taser®, etc. Things go way too fast in a crisis situation and you will probably have tunnel vision focusing only on the immediate threat to your safety.

Sufficient training can save your life. It will give you the skill and confidence needed to improve your chances of going home intact.

Self-Training

There is another kind of training that is also very helpful in being safe. It is actually self-training. This training involves looking at things in your life differently. It is about increasing your awareness of potential dangers that you may be exposed to.

I call this self-training because only you can do this for yourself. It requires developing a new mindset regarding how you see the world. It means training yourself to be aware of and fixing potential problems before they can happen, whenever possible. Being aware is not a one-time event. Rather it is a new level of personal consciousness.

Being aware of your safety requires you to develop a new set of habits to replace any poor or non-existing ones. For example, get in the habit of looking inside your vehicle before getting in to be sure no one is hiding inside of it.

Another example would be looking outside of your home to make sure everything is all right before opening the door of your home.

To improve your safety you need to first and foremost get in the habit of being aware of what is going on around you at all times. To improve your safety you need to evaluate all aspects of your life and determine where you can make improvements or get training. To improve your safety, get into the habit of training yourself to be safe. The value of this training is in your hands only.

Note: it takes approximately 30 days to develop new habits. Once you have them in place they become automatic (like the daily habit of brushing your teeth).

PROTECT YOURSELF FROM VIOLENCE

Self-Defense Seminars for Women

I strongly recommend self-defense training specially designed for women. Why? Many women have to deal with sexual assault, a different type of violence than what most men experience.

Self-defense seminars for women, if done correctly, teach the participants how to defend themselves in various real life situations. They also teach various skills such as how to call out for help and how to escape. Some of these seminars also teach women about what tools they can effectively carry and use to aid in defending themselves such as pepper spray, Kubotans, Tasers® and stun guns, etc.

For many women, these seminars are the first self-defense training that they will have ever received. These trainings are great confidence builders.

At many of these seminars men are excluded from participation and observation. Women usually find this exclusion helpful to learning as they can interact without restrictions. The only exception would be the use of a trained male to simulate attacks during parts of the training.

Self-defense seminars for women can vary in length from a few hours to several weekends, depending on the nature of the training offered.

These seminars can go a long way in showing participants what really does work versus what they thought would work.

Self-defense seminars for women are offered periodically at such places as martial arts studios, community recreation centers, the YMCA, community colleges and other locations.

Security in Your Home, Workplace & Vehicle

"Your home is your castle," or it should be. It is no accident that this saying has been around for so long. In the medieval days a castle was a fortified home for the feudal lord designed to withstand violent attacks.

Nowadays your home should still be fortified; at least enough to keep you safe from criminal attack. Just what would make your home safer? The following are some tried and true things that you can do; their viability determined by whether you live in an urban, suburban or rural environment.

Security In Your Suburban Home

First and foremost is an alarm system. These are extremely viable deterrents that can have police or security personnel at your site in minutes *if* you live close enough to these resources. This means that someone breaking in only has minutes to get in and out or to disable the alarm system. Most criminals don't have the skills to do this effectively so they will usually bug out when they hear the alarm.

The second suggestion that I have is to get a dog. Most dogs are excellent watchdogs that will bark if they sense anything is wrong and there are a number of dogs that can also effectively protect you. I would like to suggest that you get a copy of a good dog breeds' book such as *Barron's Encyclopedia of Dog Breeds*, for more information as to which breeds excel in these areas. In addition, keeping your dog in the house with you is especially effective as a deterrent. Many criminals prefer to avoid homes that have dogs.

My third suggestion is to make your home difficult to break into. Secure all windows and doors and keep them locked at all times, including those on upper stories. In the inner cities it is very common to see homes with bars on the windows and a heavy-duty metal security screen doors

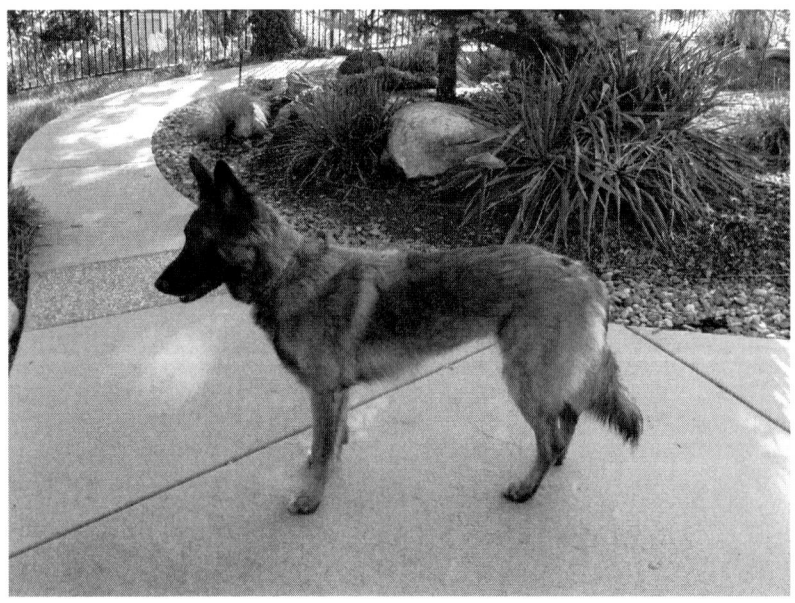

The Belgian Malinois is large, athletic and an excellent protection dog. With proper training, socialization and conditioning it can make a wonderful protection dog capable of keeping up with joggers and mountain bike riders.

in front of the solid wood or metal entryway door. They do this because of the high rate of crime. I know that many people in suburban areas won't do all of these things because of aesthetics and for not wanting to look paranoid, but you can still make other improvements in securing your home.

At the very least, I would suggest that you close and lock your doors and windows and put a wooden dowel inside your window's sliding mechanism to prevent the window from being opened or to allow only partial opening of the window. You can also install a heavy-duty pry proof front door and door jams. Heavy-duty metal front screen doors can be attractive and are being installed on many suburban

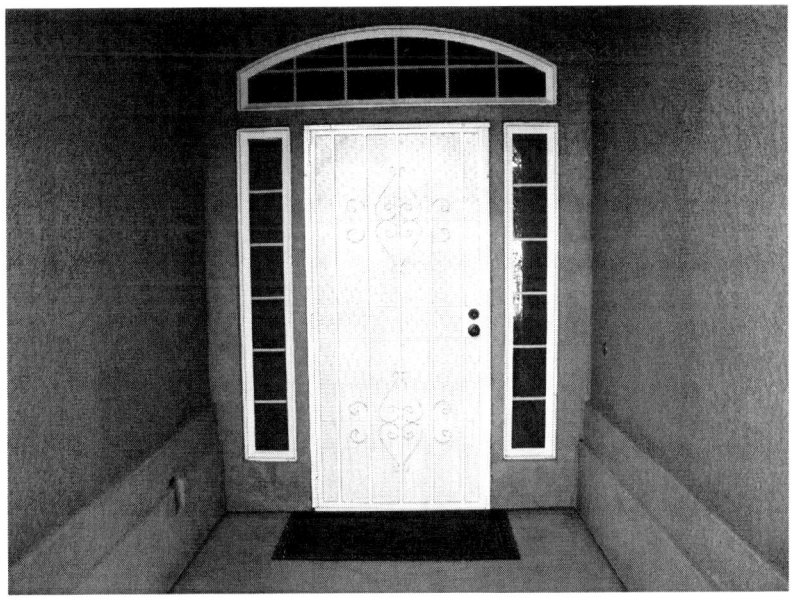

Heavy-duty decorative metal screen doors such as this are not only attractive, but can make your home significantly more resistant to forced criminal entry. Notice the metal jams around all sides of the door making forced entry very difficult.

community homes.

Fourth, if you have a yard, fence it and lock the gate.

Lastly, put thorny bushes such as roses or cacti below your windows.

For those that can't afford an alarm system or who are renting their residence, there are window and door battery operated magnetic alarms (commonly referred to as screamers). These are installed with adhesive tape and are very inexpensive (usually under $10 each at the time this book

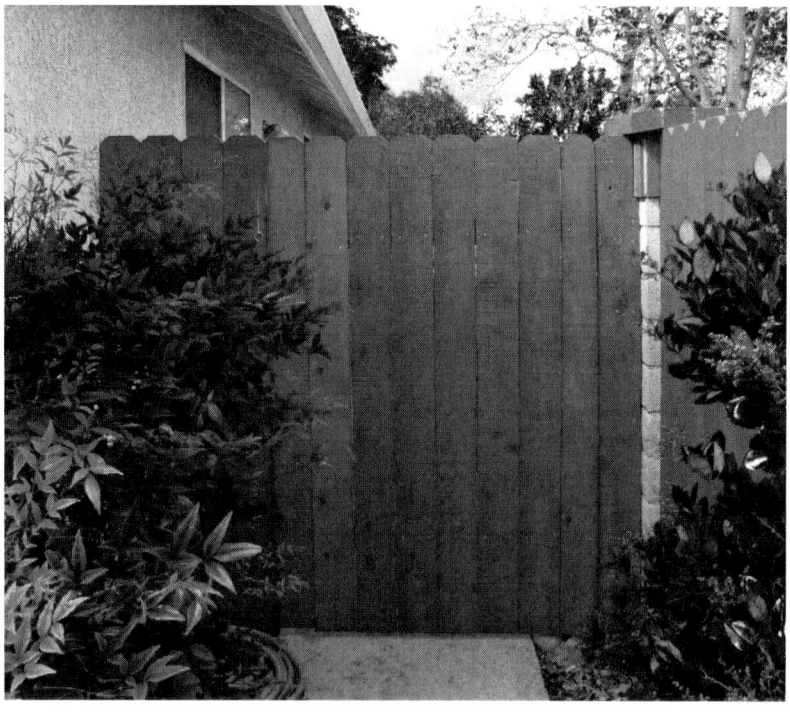

A high solid fence gate such as this makes it more difficult for criminals to see what is behind it (such as a large dog) as well as being obviously more difficult to get over.

was written). These will warn you and any nearby neighbors that someone is breaking in, and can be a good deterrent.

There are many other things that a person can do to make their home safer such as installing night lighting and cameras, and eliminating bushes and other obstructions from your yard that criminals can hide behind.

Many criminal attacks occur when someone is going in or out of their home. Always take a good look around before you head to your front door or before you go outside.

When you are home, do not unlock and open the door for anyone unless you are positive that you know that person. Period. No exceptions. If the person knocking at your door thinks you are rude for talking to them through the door, then too bad. Being safe always comes first.

Security in Your Urban Residence/Apartment

For those who live in inner-city environments with fire escapes and stairways, things can be more difficult but not impossible to secure. Watch out for young athletic criminals who work their way down fire escapes. When I lived in New York City in the 1970's, my large dog (many people who live in city apartments have large protective dogs) scared off a young man sliding down from the fire escape above onto my fire escape on a long wooden pole. Trust me, criminals can be creative. In this case, security bars on the windows that the fire escape has access to would prevent criminal entry. Make sure security bars that you put up are approved by your landlord and your local fire marshal and have quick removal for fire safety.

A heavy-duty metal door or metal reinforced door with heavy-duty locks such as a police lock and a peephole will go a long way to securing your residence. If you have a secondary access door to the hallway, make sure that it is also heavy duty. Keep both doors securely locked at all times.

And of course, an alarm system or battery operated magnetic alarms (screamers) would greatly improve your security.

Please be careful, not casual or assuming, when someone buzzes your apartment to get into your building. Make sure that you know for sure who they are before letting them in. Your building has a locked exterior door so that you will not have any undesirable persons getting inside. It is there for your security. Speak to your neighbors if you observe them letting people in without verification.

Stairways and floor lighting are also a concern in many urban buildings. They are usually dependent upon artificial lighting and can be very dark if light bulbs are out. It is not uncommon for criminals to unscrew or otherwise render them non-functional and wait in a darkened area for someone to come along who they can rob, mug or victimize in some other manner. Be especially wary if the hallway lights are out in your building.

Lastly, make sure that your roof access door is locked and remains locked at all times. It is not uncommon for criminals to gain access to a different building's rooftop and then travel from roof to roof until they get to the roof of the building that they have targeted.

GEORGE A. DEFILLIPO

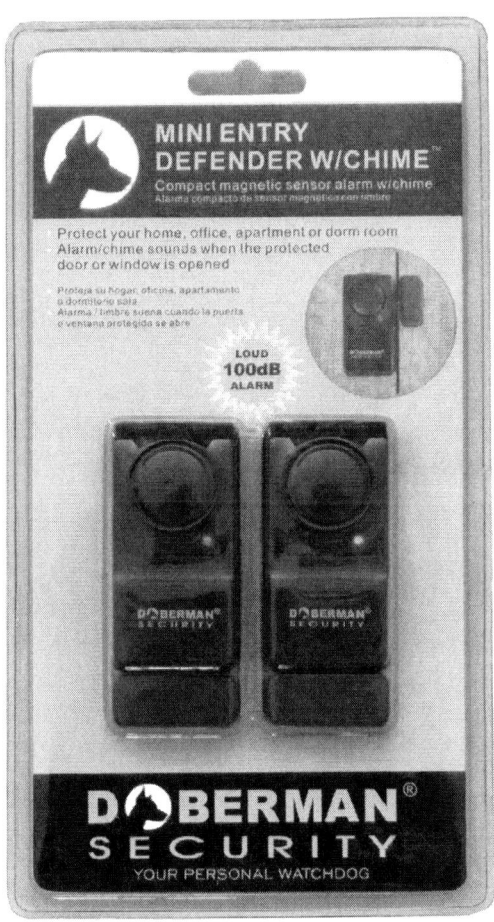

Window and door battery operated magnetic alarms (also called "screamers") are very affordable and easy to install.

Security in your Rural Home

If you live in a rural location, an alarm system probably will not be a viable option. Help is probably just too far away. Dogs are wonderful and I strongly recommend them. I recommend that you consider getting some livestock protection dogs such as the Anatolian Shepherd. They are big, hardy, athletic dogs and take guarding their charges very seriously (both your family and your livestock). They are not for everybody though, so learn more about them and decide if they would be right for you. Note: these dogs are not suitable for urban or suburban environments in most situations.

Many home invasions occur in rural areas. My suggestion is to make access to your property more difficult by installing a strong, ram-proof and bolt-cutter proof gate (like those found on federal managed lands) that is kept locked when you are not going through it. Installing fencing and a regular locked gate further away from the ram-proof gate so that those on foot cannot just walk around the gate to get access to your place is also wise. In addition, I suggest that you also consider investing in a perimeter intrusion detection system. These systems utilize various technologies and vary very much in cost. An example of a simple and affordable technology is the radio-activated product sold by the MURS Radio Company. It is good for covering a trail or entryway onto your property. I believe that many rural residents will find perimeter intrusion systems helpful in increasing the security of their property.

Having someone around who is security minded is also very helpful. Keeping firearms within reach at all times should be considered as a viable option. The further out that you live in a rural area, the less likely that someone will travel that far when there are closer rural homes around to victimize, but it is still possible. No one is totally inaccessible to criminals, even those living in the most remote locations.

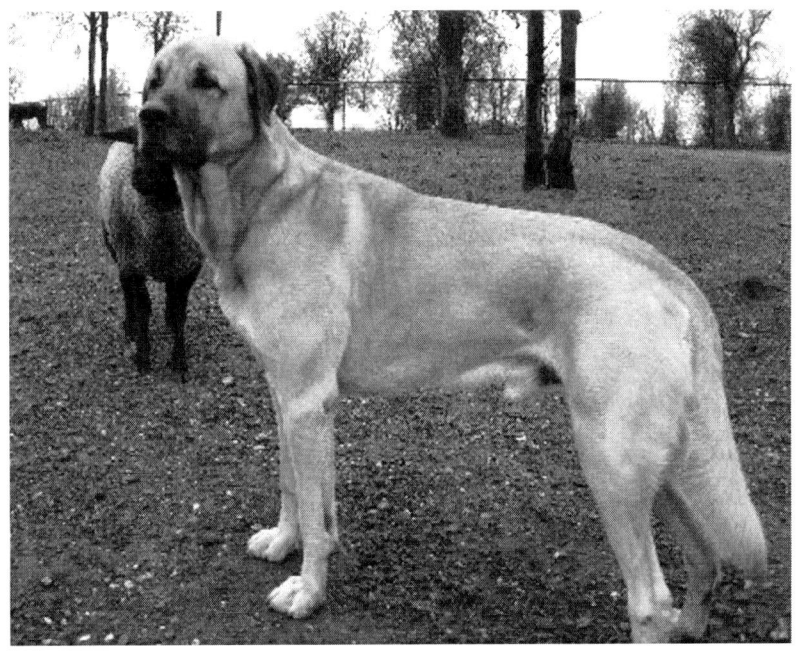

Anatolian Shepherd livestock protection dog.
Photo courtesy of Rare Breeds Ranch,
www.rarebreedsranch.com

Security At Your Workplace

A lot of what I have stated for securing your home can apply to your workplace. If you own the business you can install security cameras, alarms, secured fencing, doors that open only when a button is pushed, bulletproof partitions, have a protection dog, etc. Unfortunately, you may be forced to let strangers into your workplace because of the nature of your business or job. If so, be vigilant and armed where legal.

Exercise care when entering your place of work so that no one can sneak up on you. Be extra vigilant when leaving, especially when going to your vehicle. Many people are tired after a long day's work and put their guard down. This is not the time to do so. Wait until you get inside your secure vehicle.

Security And Your Vehicle

Be aware of anyone who may be near your vehicle or could reach your vehicle before you can. If someone starts heading toward you or your vehicle consider changing course. If possible, head to a safe public location. If you have someone heading towards you before you can get into your car or get to a safe location, then try to put something between you and that person, even if it is your car. Be ready to defend yourself.

When you reach your vehicle safely, always look inside to make sure no one is hiding inside, especially on the floor behind the seats. If safe, get into your car quickly and *lock the doors* first thing. Do not do anything else until the doors are locked. Next, *turn on the engine.* If it seems safe, you can deal with whatever else that needs your attention now, but be ready to leave quickly if need be.

Always leave enough room between your vehicle and the vehicle in front of you so that you can get past it when you stop at a red light or stop sign. That way if someone tries to approach you on foot you can drive away by driving around the other vehicle.

Try to keep an eye out for any vehicle that may be following you as you drive. If you suspect that you are being followed, *do not go straight home.* Go to a public place where there are a lot of people. Criminals will probably not follow you there. If you can, flag down a police officer.

Be especially aware of any vehicles that may be following you when you are traveling or going on vacation out of the area that you live in, especially if you go to a remote location. Travelers have been victimized while traveling through or to remote areas. Many predators will look for vehicles with out of state license plates knowing that the owners are often unfamiliar with the area that they are visiting.

Lastly, keep your car in good repair and with at least half a tank of gas. You do not want to breakdown because of a mechanical problem that could have been avoided.

Protect Yourself from Violence

Especially Dangerous Places and Situations

There are a number of places and situations that have a higher risk of people being victims of violent crime. These include some impoverished inner city areas and some social situations where conflicts between different groups of people such as gangs occur. Also, you could find yourself in a violent situation where an individual decides to randomly shoot people, frequently for no rational reason. Then there is the possibility of having to deal with widespread violence that could occur as a result of lawlessness/riots or after a natural disaster when looting is common.

Impoverished Inner City Areas

Crime is higher when people are impoverished and opportunities are diminished such as you find in many inner cities and other poor areas. I grew up and lived in these kinds of areas for many years. Most people who live in these areas are good and honest. Unfortunately, they are preyed upon by the criminal elements that live amongst them.

My life changed significantly when I moved away to a less impoverished area and it is my recommendation that people living in high crime areas consider doing likewise if they can afford to do so. If not, then my advice is to fortify your home and property. I also recommend that you be extremely careful when you go out as well as where you go. Try to minimize going out late at night when the predators are on the prowl. If you must go out late at night, then take precautions such as not going out alone. And please, only go to safe destinations.

Being aware, avoiding problems and arming oneself for self-defense situations are a part of daily survival for many people living in highly impoverished areas.

Staying out of these areas unless you have family or business there is wise. Realize that you must be extra vigilant about the possibility of criminal assault.

Social Conflicts and Gangs

When I was young there was a lot of friction between different races and ethnic groups in the impoverished areas that I lived in. Fortunately, this has diminished somewhat over the years, but it is something to still keep a look out for.

Nowadays the biggest problems in impoverished areas are with gangs. There are frequent confrontations between gangs, as well as between gang members and local residents. Gangs are constantly fighting each other whether it's over turf, drugs, apparel, colors, etc. The fighting is often brutal and deadly. In some areas, gangs control the neighborhoods.

I had a situation over twenty years ago when my nephew joined a Latino gang. He successfully recruited his brother and tried to recruit his cousin (my son). I had two choices at the time: 1) Not do anything and hope that things would work out or 2) Move far away. I chose the last and moved my family far away. This may sound extreme, however, sadly my nephew is dead now. Shot in the head execution style. He was in a coma for over two months and lived as a cripple for twelve additional years before succumbing to his injuries.

Needless to say, I made the right decision by moving and keeping my family safe. This is another example of why moving from dangerous impoverished areas is the right move for families that can manage to do so.

Shootings — Random and Otherwise

My advice is to get a concealed weapon's permit if that is an option and carry a firearm. If some lunatic, criminal or terrorist decides to start shooting people where you are, then you can defend yourself. If you can shoot that person, then you have probably saved multiple lives including your own.

I recommend getting in the habit of sitting near exits whenever possible when going to public places that have many people present. If someone starts shooting, usually the best advice is to get down quickly and work your way to the exit. Don't gawk to see what is going on. Get into survival mode as fast as humanly possible and get away.

If you cannot get away and do not have a gun, then you will have to make a personal decision about how you should handle the situation. Do you hide or do you try to stop the shooter? I cannot advise you about what to do. There are so many variables possible. I personally would want to do something if I could. And if enough people were to try to do something, there would be a chance that they could succeed.

Lawlessness

There have been many periods of lawlessness, such as riots, throughout history. Modern day examples include the 1965 Watts riot and the 1992 riot after the Rodney King police beating trial verdict. I lived in the Los Angeles area just a few miles from both riots when they occurred and was at work in Compton, California in 1992 when the verdict was announced. Let me tell you it was horrible. The school district that I worked for was closed for the duration of the riot. When it was over and we could resume educating the kids, we had to deal with a great deal of trauma first. Children should never have to be exposed to so much out of control violence and the fear that naturally is associated with it.

Many of the victims were of minority background and were randomly victimized. The gangs of the area were out of control during that riot, stealing, beating and killing people, and burning down homes and businesses. If someone left their home to get food, they were at risk of being harmed. One of the last persons killed was an elderly woman walking home with her bag of groceries.

My advice for people living in an area where riots can occur is to lie low and be ready to defend yourself at home if need be. Since riots usually last days or even a week or more, I strongly recommend maintaining a two to four week supply of food and clean water in your home at all times. Then you will not need to go out until it is all over and will have minimized the chances of something bad happening to you. Yes I know that money is often hard to come by to purchase this extra food, but if you plan properly you can acquire a little bit each week over a period of time until you have what you need.

Natural Disasters

For natural disasters such as hurricane Katrina in 2005, my advice is to leave the area before the disaster occurs if you get ample warning. If you do not get a warning, then having a supply of food and clean water, a disaster preparation kit, money and a firearm on hand can save your life. Other helpful items can include a portable water filter, a first aid kit, a portable lantern and fuel, sleeping bags for each family member, extra matches or a fire starter, a camping stove and fuel, jackets and other warm clothing, flashlights, a good knife and personal hygiene items. I recommend that everyone have at the least a two to four week supply of food and clean water on hand. Having food and clean water can allow you to sit out a disaster in a safe location. Traveling during a disaster can put you at increased risk.

Unfortunately, there are people who, during disasters, try to take advantage of others. Looting is common. Some will even work in groups to rob, rape and murder. Having a firearm is essential for your survival during these times.

As you can see, I very strongly believe that you should

make preparations to survive riots and other forms of lawlessness and natural disasters. Being able to defend yourself and your loved ones is always of critical importance regardless of the situation.

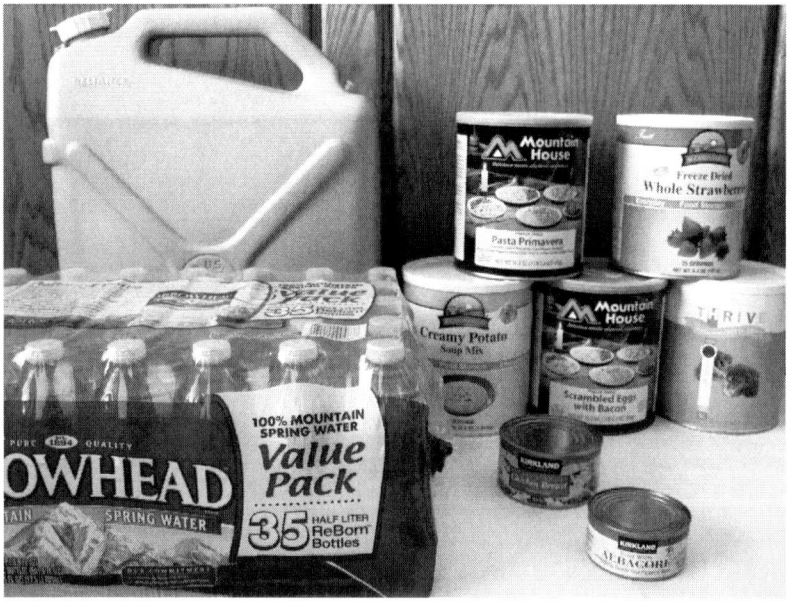

Survival emergency supply of food and water.

Legal Considerations

I would strongly suggest that anyone willing to protect himself or herself from a violent criminal attack consider finding out what weapons and other tools can be legally owned and carried in your state and city. You can look this up in your state's criminal penal codes or city's municipal codes, or you can invest a few dollars and purchase one of the guides that provides most of that information for you such as *Knife Laws of the Fifty States* and *The Traveler's Gun & Knife Law Book* by David Wong, Esq., *Traveler's Guide to the Firearm Laws of the Fifty States* by J. Scott Kappas, Esq. or *California Gun Laws* by C.D. Michel (see the Recommended Reading section for more information on this subject).

For example, California has very unfriendly gun laws with some laws being arbitrarily applied. In some counties of California you can get a permit to carry a firearm concealed if you do not have a criminal record or mental illness history. In other counties, such as Los Angeles, it is nearly impossible to get such a permit.

There are guns that are illegal to own in California that are perfectly legal to own in other states. Every state's laws on firearms are different.

When it comes to knives, California has strict laws about the concealed carry of fixed blade knives, but allows

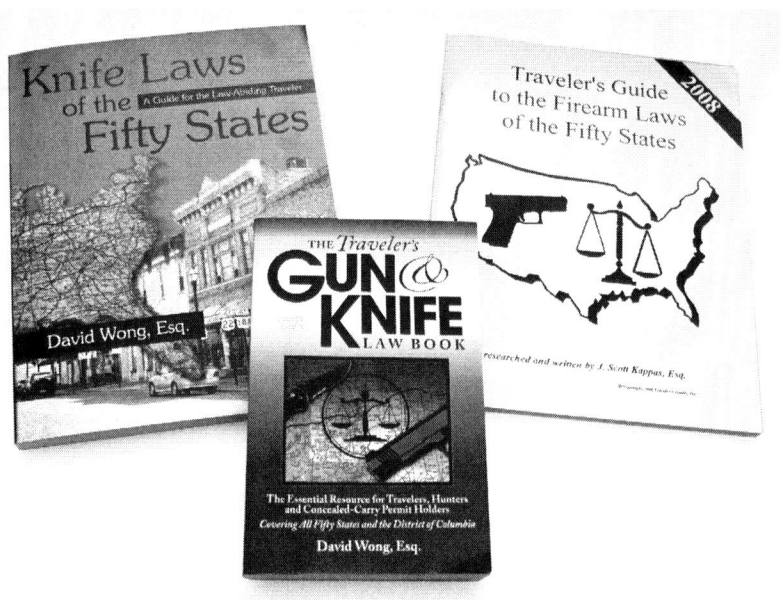

Three very useful firearm and knife law books that can help keep you legal. Bloomfield Press is a good source of books that can keep you legally informed. They can be found at gunlaws.com

closed carry of folding knives of any length except in state or local public buildings or public meetings where four-inch limits exist. Note: schools have even stricter laws regarding knives. Again, every state's laws are different and your city's municipal laws may limit blade length even further.

It is up to the reader to find out what weapon he or she can legally own and carry, as well as what limitations may exist with that weapon. It is also the reader's responsibility to stay abreast of any changes to current laws. Note: Weapons in federal buildings and facilities are typically restricted and usually prohibited.

Lastly, the law can be very tricky and the use of deadly force is justified in very limited situations (you should only use the amount of force that you need to eliminate or stop the threat). If you ever have to use deadly force, remember to politely inform the police that you need to give your statement and answer questions with an attorney present. Be especially careful what you say when calling 911 initially reporting the incident. These calls are recorded. Many people have been sent to prison because they did not follow this advice and gave a statement while they were still emotionally upset and it was used against them in a court of law.

PROTECT YOURSELF FROM VIOLENCE

How Do You Rate Being Safe?

Take a few minutes to complete this self-evaluation. It will provide you with feedback as to how well you are prepared to be safe from violence. This information is for your use only. Respond as accurately as you can and you will have a clearer idea of how safe you are and what areas that you might need to consider making improvements.

At the end is a rating scale for how you did overall.

Awareness – *Choose only one response to the following statement:*

"You look around for things that are not right."

Always	10 points
Most of the time	7 points
Occasionally	3 points
Rarely	1 point
Never	0 points

Awareness – *Give yourself one point for each of the following that applies:*

- You always look inside of your car before getting in.
- You always look outside before leaving your home, work, etc.
- You always take a good look around before leaving or going to your car.
- You look ahead, to your sides and occasionally behind you as you walk.

Avoidance – *Choose only one response to the following statement:*

"You avoid dangerous places, situations & people."

Always	10 points
Most of the time	7 points
Occasionally	3 points
Rarely	1 point
Never	0 points

Avoidance – *Give yourself one point for each of the following that applies:*

- You avoid going out late at night.
- You always take a longer route if it is safer.
- You avoid responding to negative remarks from strangers.
- You do not let strangers near you when possible.
- You quickly leave when you sense potential trouble.
- You always lock your car or home immediately upon entering.

Armed – *Choose only one response to the following statement:*
"You are armed with a gun or knife."

Always	10 points
Most of the time	7 points
Occasionally	3 points
Rarely	1 point
Never	0 points

Armed – *Give yourself one point for each of the following that applies:*

- You always have a gun available at home. (See * below)
- You always carry a knife with you.
- You always carry a Taser®, stun gun or pepper spray with you.
- You always carry more than one self-defense weapon with you.

Preparedness – *Choose only one response to the following statement:*

"You are prepared to protect yourself."

Always	10 points
Most of the time	7 points
Occasionally	3 points
Rarely	1 point
Never	0 points

Preparedness – *Give yourself one point for each of the following that applies:*
- You have an alarm system or battery operated magnetic window and door alarm devices.
- You always leave your doors locked, even when home.
- You own a large protection dog.
- You have a two to four week supply of food and water.
- You are mentally prepared to defend yourself and your family.
- You own multiple self-defense weapons.

Bonus points: raise your score an additional 10 points if you carry a firearm and have a license for concealed carry or if you live in a state where no license is legally required to do so. Carrying a firearm significantly improves the odds of not being a victim.

There were 60 points possible (70 with the bonus points).
- A score of 54 or higher (90%) means that you did superbly well and only need to keep yourself on this level or higher.
- A score of 48 to 53 (80%) means that you are in really good shape and only need a few improvements.
- A score of 42 to 47 (70%) means that you are doing pretty good, but should look at how you can improve.
- A score of 36 to 41 (60%) means that you really need to consider making improvements.
- A score of 35 or below means that you are probably vulnerable too much of the time and should consider making serious changes to lower your risk of being a victim.

Do not worry if you scored low and need to make improvements. This evaluation is just a tool to help raise your awareness so that you can make yourself safer. Remember preparations improve the odds of being safe by making you less vulnerable.

Conclusion

You have been presented with many concepts and suggestions that can be helpful in making you safer. Which ones you choose to make part of your life will depend upon your lifestyle, personal beliefs and your willingness to make changes.

For some people taking steps to be safe from violence will mean doing a number of things very differently. For others, who have already been working at being safe, it could mean just fine-tuning what you are doing. Everyone's situation is different.

Being safe is not about being paranoid, but about heightened awareness and taking sensible safeguards. You still need to go out, enjoy life and have fun. Just do it more safely.

Best wishes for a safer and more secure future.

Protect Yourself from Violence

Appendix A

Why So Many Martial Artists Oppose More Gun Control

REPRINTED BY PERMISSION OF BLACK BELT MAGAZINE/WWW.BLACKBELTMAG.COM.
(April/May 2013 issue)

For several decades – and especially after the Newtown, Connecticut, shootings – many in government and the media have called for gun control. Because firearms are an integral part of self-defense for millions of Americans, I'd like to address the issue here.

My aim is not to persuade anyone that all gun laws should be abolished or to argue that everyone should carry a gun. Rather, it's to help anti-gunners understand why their gun-carrying counterparts are up in arms and thereby eliminate some of the divisiveness that surrounds the issue.

First, those calls for gun control actually should be calls for more gun control. There are already hundreds of gun-related laws on the books. Here are a few of them.

Before 1934, it was legal to buy a full-automatic rifle or sawed-off shotgun. Remember the Tommy gun, that .45-caliber submachine gun that's in all the old gangster movies? You could get one delivered to your home. Then the

National Firearms Act was passed, and among other things, it regulated such weapons via registration and taxation. Don't bother looking up stats on how much the murder rate plunged. You won't find any.

Before 1968, it was possible to buy virtually any legal rifle or handgun through the mail – even if you were under 18. Then the Gun Control Act of 1968 was passed, and among other things, it prohibited such transactions. Does anyone remember a huge drop in crime? Me, neither.

Before 1994, it was legal to buy a semi-automatic rifle- the media prefer to use the made-up term "assault weapon" because it's scarier – with a pistol grip, bayonet lug, flash hider and removable magazines of any capacity. Then the Federal Assault Weapons Ban was passed, prohibiting certain features and limiting new magazines to 10 rounds.

Do you remember how much crime plummeted? No, because it didn't. In fact, the U.S. Department of Justice said – even as it argued in favor of the law – that there likely would be no noticeable effect on crime if the ban was renewed. After it expired in 2004, it was deemed feel-good-but-change-nothing legislation.

Now there are cries to confiscate semi-auto rifles and 30-round magazines. Here's why gun owners are upset:

Limiting a magazine to 20 rounds may sound reasonable, but it won't change a thing. It's easy to fire 20 rounds, press a button to drop the empty magazine, pop in another one and continue shooting.

The first time some lunatic does that after the proposed ban on 30-round magazines is passed, legislators will push for a 10 round limit. Don't think so? Ten rounds has been the limit in California for years. Until January 15, 2013, it was the legal limit in New York, too, but politicians there decided it was too many and rammed through a seven-round limit.

You can imagine the next step: A crime is committed, and the rhetoric revs up again: "Seven rounds is too many. We need to limit everyone to five rounds." Another crime and it goes down to three. Then one. That would mark the end of the semi-automatic rifle for self-defense.

That's fine, you may be thinking, because people would still have semi-auto handguns. Be honest here: Will banning semi-auto rifles stop crazy people from killing unarmed victims? No. They're crazy but they're not stupid. They'll use handguns, and in no time, handgun magazines will see their capacity dwindle – if it hasn't been mandated by the time you read this.

What would that leave for self-defense? Lever-action, pump action, bolt action and single-shot rifles and shotguns, along with revolvers. They'll be available – until a few homicidal maniacs use them to commit mass murder. The undeniable fact is laws won't keep mentally defective people from killing other people – only force can stop force – but that won't prevent politicians from targeting the remaining types of firearms.

Don't think so? Look at Australia. Two mass shootings there in 1987 led to the prohibition of many types of firearms – including pump action shotguns – that are capable of "rapid fire."

At some point, criminals will catch on. They'll figure out that no one is armed anymore – except themselves. That means breaking and entering homes will no longer involve risking their lives. Don't think so? Look at the U.K again, where guns are mostly banned and "hot burglaries" (crimes done when the criminals know the homeowners are present) occur at triple the rate in the USA.

That's OK, you might be thinking, because you're a skilled martial artist. Sure, you're capable of defending yourself with a club, a sword, or your hands and feet now, while you're in your prime. But what happens when you're 70? When you're 85 and in a wheelchair? When you're at work and your wife and baby are home alone? When your daughter moves into a cheap apartment near her college?

Self-defense, whether armed or otherwise, is not just the right of burly men; it's the God-given right of every human being. Fortunately for Americans, it's guaranteed by the Second Amendment, and it was upheld by the Supreme Court in 2008 and again in 2010.

But that's not stopping politicians, so let's proceed a little down the slippery slope we're on. What if a mentally disturbed person ran into a classroom, barricaded the door, pulled a sword out of his trench coat and hacked up 20 children? Sword bans could follow. Don't think so? In 2008 it became illegal in England and Wales to sell, make or import samurai swords because they were being used to commit increasing numbers of crimes.

What if a deranged man did the same thing with a bowie knife? Would knife control follow? With the right momentum, it could. Don't think so? After a man slashed 22 kids in a Chinese elementary school on December 14, 2012, the government said it would institute knife registration. And remember that in the U.K., it's pretty much illegal to carry a knife for self-defense.

What this debate needs is honesty. If politicians support

banning guns – and eventually swords, knives and all weapons – they should be honest about it. They shouldn't tell the public this *one* next law will make them safer when they know full well it won't. All it will do is take us one step closer to a defenseless population.

That, in a nutshell, is why pro-Second Amendment people are enraged – gun bans never stop. Gun-control proponents are exploiting the short attention span of the public. Otherwise, people would remember all the laws that were passed and did nothing to reduce crime.

Still, some people are OK with this. They believe a world with no weapons is possible. Maybe they think the martial arts would flourish under such conditions. They might want to think again.

It was less than a year ago when *Black Belt* Hall of Fame member Tim Larkin was prohibited from entering the U.K. Officials feared he would teach a brand of unarmed self-defense that was "not conducive to the public good."

It would seem that slope is slipperier than we thought because in some parts of the world, law-abiding citizens are already at the bottom.

Robert W. Young
Executive Editor
Black Belt Magazine

PROTECT YOURSELF FROM VIOLENCE

Appendix B

Where to Find Quality Training

Firearms

I recommend that you seek out a professional firearms instructor to learn the correct way of safely handling and accurately firing your firearms. You can contact your local gun club, shooting range or retail store for information about local instructors or you can contact the National Rifle Association, the largest source of firearms training courses in the United States, for their recommendations. You can reach the NRA at www.nra.org or call them at (703) 267-1500.

Knives and Impact Weapons

Martial arts studios and dojos often provide students with instruction in self-defense with knives and impact weapons such as sticks, canes and flashlights. Ask if they provide this training separately or if you have to enroll in their martial arts program to learn these skills as an advanced student.

Many martial arts studios also provide instruction in the Filipino martial arts of Arnis, Escrima or Kali. These arts often teach students from day one self-defense with sticks and sometimes knives.

Mace® and Pepper Spray

Some retail stores can direct you to local trainers in these chemicals for self-defense. Also, some firearms instructors are qualified to teach the use of Mace® and pepper spray. The National Rifle Association trains certified pepper spray instructors. They can be reached at www.nra.org or call them at (703) 267-1500. If all else fails, contact the manufacturers of these products for sources of training with their products. Some of these companies sell dispensers loaded with inert substances so you can practice without suffering the adverse affects of these chemicals.

Martial Arts

Your phone directory is a good source for local martial arts schools, studios and dojos. There are a number of martial arts directories on the internet that provide listings for specific cities. Although word of mouth recommendations can be helpful, you must do your own research as to which ones are best able to meet your specific self-defense needs. If possible, make an appointment with the head instructor of any schools that you may be interested in. Learn more about their system, how they teach, what is expected of students, possible contracts and costs, when classes are held, etc., before making your decision.

Tasers® and Stun Guns

Shieldher is an organization that "educates women about the benefits of personal protection with a Taser® C2." They offer Tasers® for sale as well as training for women in the use of them. They can be reached at www.Shieldher.com or by calling (602) 881-0802.

In addition, you can contact the manufacturer or retail store that you purchased your Taser® or stun gun from for information regarding other sources of training with these tools.

Glossary

Grapple: To try to seize or grasp hold of.

Ground fighting: Hand-to-hand combat which takes place on the ground. Generally it involves grappling and can involve a fighting art such as wrestling, JuJitsu, etc. Combatants frequently strike, choke or joint-lock their opponents inflicting pain and/or injury.

Impact weapons: A physical object used to strike another person. Frequently these objects extend the reach of the person using them. Most impact weapons are capable of inflicting deadly or crippling force. Common examples are the stick or baton.

Kubotan: A cylinder shaped object usually made of plastic or metal measuring 5.5" long and .56" wide. Designed to inflict controlled pain on pressure points and joints as a compliance tool for police. With keys attached, it can be used as a flailing weapon. It can be replaced with everyday items such as pens, flashlights, magic markers, etc. Invented by martial arts expert Takayuki Kubota.

Stun gun: A non-lethal tool that uses high electrical voltage (with low amperage) to incapacitate an attacker. It must be held against the attacker's body to be effective. There are many models sold that vary in their voltage capacity.

Taser®: An electrical device that operates similarly to the stun gun except that it shoots its electrical probes through the air onto an attacker via attached wires in order to incapacitate.

Recommended Reading

Dogs

D. Caroline Coile, Ph.D.
Encyclopedia of Dog Breeds
Barron's Educational Series, Inc.
Hauppauge, NY   2005
(*Informative coverage of dog breeds.*)

Orysia Dawydiak & David Sims
Livestock Protection Dogs
Alpine Blue Ribbon Books
Loveland, Colorado   2004
(*A valuable source of information on dog breeds used for livestock protection.*)

Richard Beauchamp
Anatolian Shepherd Dog
Kennel Club Books
Allenhurst, New Jersey   2006
(*Good specific information about this breed.*)

Guns

J. Scott Kappas, Esq.
*Traveler's Guide to the Firearm
Laws of the Fifty States*
Traveler's Guide, Inc.
Covington, Kentucky   2008
(*Helpful information about various state laws for someone traveling with firearms.*)

C.D. Michel, attorney at law
California Gun Laws
COLDAW Publishing
Long Beach, CA   2012/2013
(*A very useful guide to California's state and Federal firearms regulations.*)

Massad F. Ayoob
*In The Gravest Extreme:
The Role of the Firearm in Personal Protection*
Police Bookshelf
P.O. Box 122
Concord, New Hampshire   1980
(*The definitive work on the use of deadly force. A must read for CCW permit holders.*)

National Rifle Association
The Basics of Personal Protection
Fairfax, VA   1988
(*A very good guide to the basics of self-protection with a handgun.*)

Guns and Knives

David Wong, Esq.
The Traveler's Gun & Knife Law Book
Spartan Press, L.L.C.
Nashua, New Hampshire   2010
(*Helpful information about various state gun and knife laws.*)

Knives

David Wong, Esq.
Knife Laws of the Fifty States
AuthorHouse
Bloomington, IN   2006
(*An excellent guide to knife laws.*)

Bill Bagwell
*Bowies, Big Knives, and the Best
Of Battle Blades*
Paladin Press
Boulder, Colorado   2000
(*Makes a strong argument for why a properly designed Bowie knife is the superior fighting knife. Good information on other knife designs.*)

John Sanchez
Blade Master
Paladin Press
Boulder, Colorado   1983
(*A classic on survival skills for fighting with a knife. Good illustrations.*)

John Sanchez
Slash and Thrust
Paladin Press
Boulder, Colorado   1980
(*More good information about fighting with a knife.*)

John Styers
Cold Steel
Paladin Press
Boulder, Colorado   1952
(*Good explanation/pictures of military hand-to-hand combat with knives and other weapons.*)

Martial Arts

Black Belt Magazine
Black Belt
Communications, LLC
An Active Interest Media Publication
24900 Anza Dr. Unit E
Valencia, CA 91355
(*A premier martial arts publication.*)

Remy Presas
Modern Arnis
Ohara Publications
Santa Clarita, CA   1983
(*Explains the Filipino art of stick fighting. Good photos.*)

Takayuki Kubota & John G. Peters, Jr.
Official KUBOTAN Techniques
Reliapon Police Products
Albuquerque, New Mexico   1983
(*This book is a very good supplement to Kubotan training classes.*)

Lawrence Kane & Kris Wilder
How To Win A Fight
Gotham Books
New York, NY   2011
(*Overall, good advice on how to avoid getting into a fight and what to do if you can't.*)

Prof. Jane Carr, Geri Copitch, Robert Sedillos, Philip Copitch
Anatomy For Martial Artists
Hutzpah Press
Igo, CA   2011
(*An anatomy guide by martial artists for martial artists. Excellent illustrations.*)

Scott Redden
Opening Your Mind With Martial Arts
Self-published
P.O. Box 494279
Redding, CA   2012
(*Insights of the Filipino martial art of Arnis with good general self-defense information.*)

Self Protection

Massad Ayoob
The Truth About Self Protection
Police Bookshelf
P.O. Box 122
Concord, New Hampshire   1983
(*Excellent information about protecting yourself from criminal attacks.*)

SURVIVAL

Dave Black
Survival Retreats
Skyhorse Publishing
New York, NY   2011
(*Very good information on securing and protecting your home and yourself.*)

John "Lofty" Wiseman
SAS Urban Survival Handbook
Skyhorse Publishing
New York, NY   2008
(*Covers most every possible contingency by a former trainer of Britain's famous Special Air Service unit.*)

Jim Cobb
Prepper's Home Defense
Ulysses Press
Berkeley, CA   2012
(*Good information about protecting your family by any means necessary from a prepper's perspective.*)

James Wesley Rawles
How To Survive The End Of The World As We Know It
Penguin Group Publishing
New York, N.Y.   2009
(*A National bestseller survivalist book with excellent information on home security and self-defense.*)

About the Author

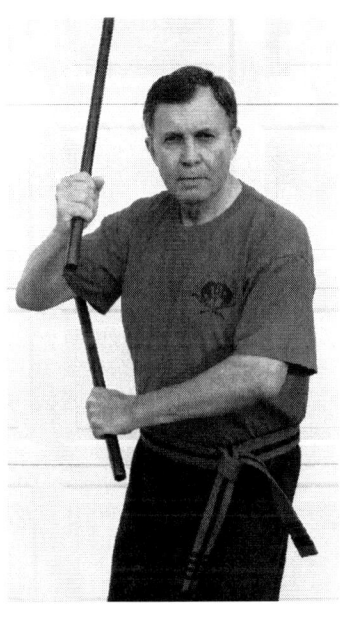

George DeFillipo has lived in some very rough and dangerous inner city areas of the United States including Bedford Stuyvesant, New York; Chicago, Illinois; Cleveland, Ohio; and Lawndale, California. All of these areas have been or are still well known for their everyday violence. While growing up and during his early adult years in the 1950's to 1970's, he had to learn to survive with his fists and his brains. Street fights and personal survival were the norms for the author during this period of time. He had no choice but to learn what it took to survive.

As an adult, the author pursued an education and the American dream. He was able to live in nicer middle class areas where violence was the exception and not the norm. Self-defense was no longer an immediate survival need, but something that he pursued for personal knowledge. He engaged in a lifetime study of fighting arts and for the last two decades has trained in the Filipino martial art of Arnis.

In addition, the author has had extensive experience with firearms, and has competed successfully in many local shooting matches.

The author sees many middle class communities experiencing increases in violence, especially since the economic downturn of 2008. It is his wish to share some of his knowledge and experience, not just with those living in inner cities, but also with those now having to deal with it as an everyday reality for the first time. It is the author's wish that the reader be provided with the information needed that will help minimize him or her becoming a victim.

The author is a retired school administrator and martial arts instructor.